ACNE
FREE FROM PIMPLES IN 7 STEPS

The path to treating acne and pimples

Francesco Antonaccio MD
(Translation by Francesca Mura)

Copyright © 2017 Francesco Antonaccio - All rights reserved

This book is protected under copyright law.
Duplication or usage for reproduction without the explicit authorization is prohibited.

Editor: CreateSpace

ISBN-13: 978-1979273336

ISBN-10: 1979273332

First edition: October 2017

WARNINGS

The information in this book is for educational purposes and to be used for guidance only.

The therapies and treatments for acne should always be tailored to the individual patient and based on the skin type and form of acne. Indeed, the treatments vary from patient to patient and so do the results, which inevitably depend on the individual response of the patient. For this reason, considering that it is not possible to guarantee the desired results following treatments given by your doctor or dermatologist, it is even less possible to guarantee the expected results simply following the advice and general information found in this book.

Before choosing any therapy, treatment, or advice, please consult your doctor. The diagnosis and treatment of acne should be respectively made and prescribed by your doctor, who will also tailor and base them on your clinical picture.

The content provided in this book should not be used for diagnostic or therapeutic purposes for acne disease or any other disease, physical condition or skin imperfection.

The author and the editor do not take any responsibility for the results or negative effects that might be caused by the use or misuse of the information contained in this book.

SUMMARY

INTRODUCTION

As a dermatologist, I have dedicated many years of my career treating acne and assessing the results of the treatments.

More than ten years ago, following my passion for cosmetology and writing, I founded the website www.dermatologiacosmetologica.it and the Facebook page Dermatologia Cosmetologica, where I write about acne and wrinkles, and interact with my readers.

Both online and in my studio I have heard (too) many stories: some patients who were desperately looking for miraculous remedies for acne, others who came across expensive or wrong treatments, and even some who abandoned the treatments altogether.

I experienced first-hand the frustration and the pain of those who were seeing their face affected by acne and still had found a way to defeat the pimples, but also those who rediscovered the joy of living as the conditions of their skin improved week by week thanks to my treatments.

I have always found fulfilment and satisfaction in helping those who suffer from acne, both on a human and professional level.

I have always acknowledged the importance of aesthetics, as well as the psychological impact that diseases of the skin and alterations have on us all, teamed with the role of cosmetology: the science of health and skin rebalance.

Since I love simplicity and have little patience myself, I have designed therapies which not only are easy to follow on a regular basis, but also rapidly give visible results. Unfortunately, for many reasons, the majority of skin conditions are persistent and chronic, and acne is no exception. During the years, I have become more and more convinced that acne disease tends to last for a long time when it is not treated effectively and, above all, when it is not faced with a more global approach. The patient needs to be taught to combine dermatologic and cosmetic therapies with a healthier diet and lifestyle.

As the acne condition improves thanks to the dermatological treatments, the patient's diet and lifestyle can and should hold an important role in the phase of stabilisation and normalisation.

Here is why I have decided to write this book.
This book is for those who suffer from acne or want to help their children who feel uncomfortable due to pimples. Its goal is to let the reader understand how to treat acne.

This book is based on what is often missing when it comes to treating acne: a global and methodical approach.

This book will teach you, step by step, why and how the pimples appear, what are the available treatments and the fundamentals of an anti-acne therapy which truly works, and finally, how to intervene in many factors in order to fight them effectively and obtain long-lasting benefits.

This book will provide you with a guide and a path to follow, establishing halfway stages and setting up a strategy to defeat acne.

Please bear in mind: I am not going to present any miraculous treatments or products!

Everything you will read is just based on a method which is simple, practical, and therefore, effective.

Following the suggestions explored in this book, you will learn how to:

- Rapidly improve your skin's condition
- Progressively eliminate blackheads and pimples
- Avoid holes and marks on your skin caused by pimples
- Progressively prevent the growth of new pimples
- Reduce the visibility of acne scars
- Maintain your skin's smoothness and cleanliness over time

Since everyone responds subjectively to therapies and is, in the end, responsible for the implementation of the treatments, it is difficult and rather impossible for a doctor to guarantee specific results. However, in this book, you will find a personal summary of my studies and clinical experiences.

The articles and research on given aspects and mechanisms of acne sometimes lead to conflicting results, and dermatologists (the skin specialists) can therefore have different opinions in this regard.

Some of my colleagues might even disagree on the information that I am going to discuss in this book.

In the past, there were many prejudices and legends about the causes of acne and its treatments. It was thought that acne and pimples were an issue related to adolescence and that "they would disappear with age".

Therefore, acne had to be accepted, passively, without a single treatment – even though the disease was disfiguring the skin and causing great psychological insecurities whose effects often undermined adult age.

Due to these erroneous certainties, i.e. "The pimples will go away" "There is nothing you can do", effective treatments had never been developed in the past. Furthermore, cosmetology was not as advanced as it is today and the treatment of acne scars was not even taken into consideration.

Everything has changed now!

There are ways to fight pimples, indeed: dermocosmetic treatments for at-home use, drugs, and dermatological treatments given at clinics.

Even the wrong popular beliefs and legends on acne have been gradually revised and corrected – although they often persist.

Why still wait?

The biggest mistake you can make is to undertake "a DIY anti-acne treatment" based on your friends' advice, your mother's advice, or other people who might not be experts – even though they have the best intentions.

As you will read in this book, an essential rule is that you should not try and follow advice untidily, but rather apply an appropriate treatment method and follow it with determination.

Whilst treating my patients with acne, I saw some of them improving rapidly, while others gradually changing: this is normal because everyone responds to treatments differently.

Some patients experienced relapses, while others permanently eliminated the skin condition. Why? How did they do it? Is it only a matter of therapy or individual response? Is there another factor involved? A different personal approach? A different lifestyle?

Is it really possible to eliminate pimples?

In the short-term, it is possible to obtain improvements with traditional anti-acne treatments, but it is better to reason strategically regarding the long-term. Unfortunately, we cannot fight the acne in a few days and, probably, not even in a few weeks.

The path that we need to take not only involves dermatological treatments, but also gets to the bottom of the root causes. It acts in depth on motivation and behaviours, nutrition and lifestyle, and all the external and internal factors able to trigger the formation of pimples on skin which is already genetically predisposed to acne.

The most recent research on epigenetics, the study of the external environment influence on our genetic heritage, say that there are factors able to shape and change (both negatively and positively) our genes activity and that, if we act selectively on these factors, it is possible to modify both the chances of healing and the disease.

Nothing is set in stone, even the genetic predisposition to acne is not an inevitable destiny: we can reduce it!

Keeping your skin as clean and healthy as possible is also a matter of habits and lifestyle: this is why method, regularity, and determination are needed.

The aim is to be free from pimples.

And in this book, I will explain to you what steps are necessary to achieve this aim.

You will be surprised, but you will see that, if you follow the principles illustrated here, you will reach a point where your pimples will continuously improve and you will soon be able to defeat acne – or at least, keep it under control.

Think about it, pimples are often a cause of discomfort and insecurity.

Following the described 7 steps, you can finally make your look and your life better!

However, it is up to you to apply this method day by day – it is the only way to do it, if you want to obtain beneficial results.

Lastly, I tried not to make the text dense, with a medical language that is too specialised; although some scientific data is necessarily present, it is written in the easiest way possible.

They are the fundamentals needed for you to understand how to act.

I hope this book will be helpful to you, inspire you and motivate you to finally fight pimples and therefore push you to do something important and significant for you and your life.

Francesco Antonaccio, MD

HOW TO USE THIS BOOK

Let this book be your guide to fight pimples in a very effective way.

This book describes a "method" which, if it is applied correctly, will allow you to increase your determination and your ability to face acne in a global and strategic way.

Its contents are divided into two parts.

In the first part, which is more theoretical but not less important, I will explain in depth how and why pimples form, the primary and secondary causes.

You will see that there are many factors involved; some of them are more controllable than others. But do not feel discouraged: it is, indeed, necessary to understand all the mechanisms concerned and their role in the manifestation of this unsightly skin condition.

This is also why you need to follow a path: step by step, it will help you face all these factors, achieve the intermediate aims and reach the final goal.

In the second part, which is more practical, I will describe the path that we will follow together and the single steps to take: you will encounter tests and assessments that will allow you to understand where you are in relation to the final goal, help you to increase your willpower so that you will not give up or fall behind the schedule. These steps will require a great open-mindedness and total participation from your side, although you might often doubt or think that some excerpts have nothing to do with the treatment of pimples.

Please, do not be doubtful or sceptical. Even the first steps will be crucial; they will let you reflect on your behaviours and gradually change your habits, leading you to improve your look and skin's condition, and to a new phase of your life.

As you will read along, you will learn why the effect of each step will make the effects of the next steps stronger.

In order to have a general overview of this book, I advise you to read it once quickly. You will then need to read it again more slowly, chapter by chapter, if you want to deepen and apply the method.

PART I

OILY SKIN

The first fundamental concept I want you to know is that **oily skin is a hereditary characteristic**, and is the basic condition for which acne can manifest.

Actually, there are 3 different situations:

1. Oily skin without pimples
2. Oily skin with occasional pimples
3. Oily skin with severe or mild acne

There are people with oily skin who have many blackheads and pimples that form regularly all over the face and, sometimes, even on breasts and back: this is a case of true acne, i.e. a skin condition of chronic course.

There are also cases of oily skin with sporadic formation of pimples, but this cannot be considered as acne.

Lastly, there are people with oily skin that have never (or very sporadically) seen pimples forming on their skin.

Despite sharing the same basic condition of oily skin, why are there differences? This is a question that will be answered in this book.

First observation: it is possible to have oily skin without having acne!

Please bear in mind: **oily skin is always prone to acne!**
Therefore, acne is always lying in wait.
Before we delve into this book further and learn more about acne, we should question ourselves on some concepts and clear our ideas by making a few distinctions between "having acne", "having oily skin", and "having normal skin".

When acne is eliminated, will you finally have a "normal skin"?
Of course you won't!
And how do we define normal skin? Skin with a normal sebum secretion, which is neither oily nor dry, a middle way?
It is a very rare circumstance.

It might be better to consider normal skin as an ideal state of perfect balance. The concept of normal skin is a little deceptive because it often indicates a rather theoretical and abstract situation, which corresponds to a healthy, beautiful and perfect looking skin: a top model's skin.

The truth is that no one can always have a normal skin.

The skin, even when it appears healthy and "normal", is in a state of dynamic and precarious balance.

But let us go back to focus on oily skin, a more frequent and real condition.

HOW TO RECOGNISE OILY SKIN

Let us consider the characteristics of oily skin.

If you train yourself to observe them, you will be able to perform a self-assessment of the skin and understand (indicatively) if your skin is in fact oily, and how oily it is.

Subjective sensation:
- 0, itch, burning

To the touch:
- greasy, thick
- solid, smooth

To the eye:
- rosy, red, greenish
- shiny, grainy, dilated pores
- microcomedones
- finely desquamating

In my professional practice as dermatologist, I have noticed that patients are often very aware of having oily skin because they see that it is shiny and feels greasy.

In some cases, which are even rather frequent, patients think they have dry skin – so dry that they feel the need to apply hydrating products.

They actually have asphyxiated skin or apparently mixed, which is nothing more than a variant of oily skin.

As you will read later in book, this is a major evaluation mistake which can cause a rather sudden and persistent form of acne.

A further distinction to make is that oily skin, in some areas of the face, can be thicker and appear opaque instead of shiny, and rough instead of oily to the touch.

THE CHARACTERISTICS OF MIXED OR ASPHYXIATED SKIN

According to the self-assessment of the skin, we can see how mixed or asphyxiated skin is characterised:

Subjective sensation:
- 0, itch

To the touch:
- rough, smooth
- dry, greasy

To the eye:
- grey-yellowish
- opaque
- shiny just in the T-zone (but not always)
- grainy
- dilated pores and microcomedones
- desquamating

Many characteristics (except those indicated in italics) match those of oily skin.

The rule is that, if dilated pores and microcomedones are present, it is always oily skin prone to acne.

IS ACNE ALWAYS JUVENILE?

By definition, acne is juvenile, linked to puberty and adolescence.

But is this always true? Not really. I know this is not good news, but I have to debunk a myth that I was mentioning in the introduction.

We have seen that oily skin is prone to form comedones and pimples, and – another important concept – this predisposition tends to persist until adult age.

For instance, this is the case of women who have oily skin, but only a few blackheads and whiteheads, and little sporadic pimples when they were aged between 12 and 25.

Once they turn 35, they start using a hydrating or anti-wrinkles cream and after a few weeks, they have their face covered with blackheads and whiteheads, from which many pimples will progressively form.

It is normal that the patient is surprised and also frustrated.

"How come? When I was young, I only had few little pimples. I only had few blackheads, but I have never had acne!"

We are facing a case of cosmetic acne, in a patient with skin prone to acne who thought she only had slightly oily skin and spent her young age unharmed.

Although you do not have or you have never had acne, it is important to realise that you have skin prone to acne for 2 reasons:

a.   avoiding the mistake of applying unsuitable cosmetics (as you will see in step V);
b.   utilising specific cosmetics.

In conclusion, acne is defined as 'juvenile' because it affects 80% of adolescents and there is a reason for this – as I will explain later.

But pimples can also suddenly appear in young adults.

ACNEIC OILY SKIN

Imagine you step back to your more or less recent past, to the beginning of your adolescence, when you were aged between 11 and 14.

You might have started noticing that your skin, once normal, smooth, and dry, was becoming more and more oily and shiny – "dirty".

The increase of sebum secretion, i.e. the production of skin fat (sebum), was the first sign: with the body development, there has been an increase in the production and secretion of male hormones in the blood: testosterone, androstenedione, and dehydroepiandrosterone. If you think about it, there have also been other changes in your body during that time.

And, probably, you were not even giving weight to the changes of your skin until you started feeling it rough on your nose, chin, and forehead and then, in front of the mirror, noticed the presence of **blackheads and whiteheads**, like grains of sand.

HOW A PIMPLE FORMS

Know your enemy before fighting
Sun Tzu (military strategist)

Each problem and each situation has one or more critical point on which we can act to solve them. The first step to face a problem is to understand it in depth.

We cannot eliminate acne, or improve it and keep it under control without knowing the causes and multiple aspects of this skin condition.

It is only with this knowledge that we will be able to find a global strategy, which lies at the fundamentals of the approach that I want to share with you in this book.

Let us see together how the pathology of acne develops and evolves:

why and how a pimple forms.

THE 4 MAIN FACTORS

There are four main factors that influence the development of acne.
They also explain very well the evolution from comedo to pimple.
Here they are in brief:

1.   Hormones and hyper sebum secretion
2.   Hyperkeratosis and obstruction of pilosebaceous follicles
3.   Inflammation
4.   Bacterial growth

The first two factors are crucial for triggering the pathological
process.

As we will later see, the other two: inflammation of follicles and
bacterial growth are consequences of the first ones, further amplifying
the development of acne.

It all starts from the hormones creating favourable conditions, but
if the follicle was not obstructed and the comedo did not form,
bacterial growth and inflammation would not be there.

FACTOR I: HORMONES AND HYPER SEBUM SECRETION

With adolescence, there is an increase of male sex hormones secretion and their presence in the blood.

This happens to both males and females.

In the former, the production of the main male sex hormones (testosterone) happens in the testicles; in the latter, it happens in the ovaries. In both of them, the adrenal gland produces secondary male hormones (androstenedione and dehydroepiandrosterone), but they are no less important as later they will become testosterone.

The male hormones arrive to the skin and stimulate the sebaceous glands to produce more sebum. This explains why acne affects adolescents more.

Except in those less frequent cases where there are disorders in the endocrine glands, the amount of male hormones is normal in both males and females.

In the latter, the most frequent endocrine disorder can be polycystic or micro-polycystic ovary: as we will see later, there can be an increase of male hormones produced by ovaries, and therefore, an increase of their levels in the blood and a greater stimulus of sebaceous glands.

The consequence is a more severe acne than the one that a person would "normally" have if hormone levels were normal.

Compared to females, males have obviously higher male hormone levels, and this explains why the acne is generally more evident.

If hormones represent the first cause in all adolescents, the right questions to ask are:

Why does acne only affect 80% of adolescents and not everyone?
Why do some people not suffer from acne?
If hormone levels are normal, why is acne only severe in some cases?

It is all receptors' fault!

All hormones are "messages" between cells from tissues and organs: they send activating or blocking signals to the receptors to the receptors found in the cells themselves.

Receptors are like locks, while hormones are the keys: there is a right key for each lock and vice versa.

In the sebaceous glands cells, there are specific receptors for male hormones which therefore stimulate the production of sebum.

If the receptors are very sensitive to the correspondent hormones, the stimulus (activation or block) is greater.

The receptors sensitivity is genetically determined and this explains why the pimples are more severe in some people and why there is a kind of genetic predisposition to acne.

It is then important to evaluate if parents and grandparents had acne and how severe it was.

In conclusion, hormones are important because they trigger an increase of sebum secretion, but their sole action, do not explain how pimples form.

They can explain the severity of acne, though!

Polycystic ovary: an issue not to be underestimated

In women, acne is often associated to micro-polycystic ovary. Around 10-20% of women in fertile age are affected by polycystic ovary syndrome, with scarce or absent ovulation.

Ovarian polycystosis is due to an ovarian dysfunction with a consequent increase of male hormone production by the ovary itself.

Polycystic ovary can already appear during adolescence through different manifestations: irregular menstrual cycles, infertility, signs of hirsutism (excessive hair growth in the face), acne, alopecia (hair thinning and loss), overweight or obesity, diabetes tendency, and metabolic syndrome.

Women with polycystic ovary, though, very often have irregular menstrual cycle and pimples only: this is why the dermatologist is the first person to be consulted. When dealing with a young woman with acne, the dermatologist should suspect the presence of polycystic ovary and ask her if her menstrual cycles are regular or not, checking if there is any excess of hair growth or hair loss.

In order to make an accurate diagnosis, the collaboration of the gynaecologist is crucial. During the gynaecological examination, it is possible to perform a simple non-invasive examination: the ultrasound.

There are two types of ultrasound that can be performed: abdominal and transvaginal. The latter allows performing a more accurate evaluation and the detection of ovarian cysts. When these are very small, they will lead to the diagnosis of micro-polycystic ovary – the most frequent and minor case.

If there are signs of hirsutism, the gynaecologist can prescribe hormone dosages: estrogens, progesterone, testosterone, androstenedione, dehydroepiandrosterone, and others. In this way, the entire status of male and female hormones can be evaluated.

In the case of a minor polycystic ovary, the prescribed dosages can be slightly different; this is why I personally advise to perform ultrasound first.

The first objective of the therapy is to "put ovaries at rest" with the prescription of an estrogen-progestin birth-control pill, i.e. female sex hormones which make the ovaries "sleep" and reduce the hormonal secretion by simulating a pregnancy.

This leads to 2 benefits:

1. decrease of male hormone production with reduction of sebum secretion and pimples after 3 months therapy. A greater effect can be obtained when the estrogen-progestin birth-control pill is combined with an active principle which is able to neutralise the androgen hormones action: cyproterone acetate. This can help, but it is not enough to keep pimples under control. In order to treat acne, even when it is linked to cystic ovary, dermatological and dermocosmetic anti-acne treatments must be applied.
2. slow and gradual decrease of ovarian cysts and micro-cysts until they disappear completely (generally in 1 to 3 years).

It is important to know that birth-control pill, like any other drug, has side effects and contraindications.

Therefore, before taking it, it is always necessary to:

- listen to your gynaecologist's opinion
- carry out specific laboratory examinations in order to avoid a predisposition to severe side effects. These should be repeated periodically.

In moderate cases, when acne is accompanied by evident hirsutism, androgenic alopecia and overweight, adolescent patients feel that their female image is damaged and suffer psychologically (depression and anxiety).

In severe cases, when diabetes, metabolic syndrome (hypercholesterolemia, etc.) or other hormone disorders are involved, an endocrinologist or internist should also be called out for evaluation and patient management.

In these cases, indeed, the approach should be interdisciplinary, with the collaboration between a dermatologist, gynaecologist, family doctor, endocrinologist, psychologist, and nutritionist.

In any case of acne and polycystic ovary, diet is very important and I always advise that one follows an anti-acne diet – I will talk about this later.

FACTOR II: OBSTRUCTION OF PILOSEBACEOUS FOLLICLES

Acne manifestations are characterised by a main anomaly: **ductal hyperkeratosis**, i.e. the thickening of pilosebaceous follicles duct.
This is the heart of the problem called acne!
A possible and probable consequence is the partial or total obstruction of the pore!

Why does this thickening happen?
Because the cells of the stratum corneum accumulate and stratify more.

What happens?
The stratum corneum is the outermost layer of the skin consisting of dead cells that have migrated outward from the basal layer.
The multiplication of epidermal cells (keratinocytes) normally happens for a natural process of skin renewal to replace dead cells.
This accelerates when there is an inflammatory stimulus.
In this case, the stimulus is due to the heavy production of free radicals caused by altered and excess sebum oxidation.
Skin cells start to multiply more intensely, increasing their number and, consequently, the stratum corneum thickens: here we have hyperkeratosis.

COMEDONAL ACNE
How comedones form.

Black and whiteheads are also called, respectively, open and closed comedones.

The former are more superficial and appear just as dilated pores filed with a dark substance. If you squeeze them with your fingers, this substance composed of dead cell debris and oxidised sebum (that is why it is dark) is pushed out: the pore can remain open and dilated, appearing like a minuscule hole.

Big blackheads usually indicate a greater predisposition to a more severe form of acne with nodules, cysts, and possible acne scars.

Closed comedones or whiteheads are deeper. Squeezing them is basically useless; they actually cause damage: we will see why later.

The presence of whiteheads means that the acne will worsen and that many pimples will appear in the next weeks!

Many years ago, I was explaining to one of my patients how pimples form and I really like the definition that she gave to comedones: "Closed comedones are like time bombs that, soon or later, will explode on my face". I often use it to explain that they represent the main problem of acne.

I was in my office days ago, and I was explaining to my patient how whiteheads form and how to treat them. My patient surprised me with another effective definition, but less "dramatic" than the previous one: "Whiteheads are like seeds of weed that will soon germinate and fill the field, ruining it."

In fact, let us think about it. If whiteheads did not form, acne would not exist! This is a very, very important point from the perspective of the therapy, which will be explained in depth later.

But how and why do blackheads and whiteheads form?

As previously mentioned, the first change (perfectly normal and physiological) is the increase in levels of male hormones stimulating the skin's sebaceous glands to produce more sebum.

These glands are localised in the innermost layer of the skin (into the dermis), near the hair follicle. They are cluster- shaped and have an excretory duct where the sebum passes through the hair follicle, for this reason they are known as pilosebaceous follicle.

Sebum is a very important factor in the development of acne, but it is not the only one, as we will see shortly.

Once again, a given increase in the sebum secretion is perfectly normal and occurs in all of us during puberty because of the increasing levels of male hormones.

However, in individuals with oily skin and acne, there are two issues regarding the sebum:

1. quantity (hyperproduction)
2. quality (a greater amount of free fatty acids which readily oxidise when in contact with oxygen, forming free radicals).

Now it is the time to deepen our knowledge of sebum and its functions.

Sebum is produced by the sebaceous gland connected to the follicular duct, where they pour this oily mass that will become part of the hydrolipidic film.

As the term itself suggests, **the hydrolipidic film** is like a film on the skin surface formed by a hydrophilic or aqueous component (NMF) and a fat component, composed of **sebum** (95% of the total) and epidermal lipids produced by keratinocytes.

The function of the hydro-lipid film is to prevent the evaporation and loss of water and keep the skin well hydrated. Moreover, it has antimicrobial properties due to the acidic pH and the presence of fatty acids from which toxic substances form for the bacteria. These molecules are lipoperoxides, free radicals.

The sebum composition is slightly different from person to person and contributes to the personal and characteristic smell of the body.

Composition of human sebum:

- Squalene 10%
- Paraffin 5%
- Triglycerides 35%
- Waxes 20%
- Free fatty acids 20%
- Cholesterol 10%

From this list, we can see that the human sebum is mainly composed of triglycerides, then wax, squalene, cholesterol and free fatty acids.

In particular, free fatty acids oxidise when in contact with atmospheric oxygen, forming free radicals: molecules with irritating and inflammatory properties.

Free radicals are highly reactive molecules, i.e. they react with all the other nearby substances by causing their oxidation. Once oxidised, they also become free radicals: this is a chemical chain reaction that would not cease to extend (just like a fire), if antioxidants did not intervene as "firemen", switching it off and blocking it.

The sebum of people with acne contains a higher amount of free fatty acids; for this reason, there is a greater production of free radicals near the outlet of the pilosebaceous follicle (pore) and on the skin surface. This means a higher level of inflammation and irritation!

In fact, it is precisely the inflammation from free radicals which causes the ductal hyperkeratosis: the thickening of the stratum corneum (the outermost layer of the epidermis consisting of dead cells) at the level of the upper part of the pilosebaceous follicle and, consequently, a progressive narrowing and occlusion of the pore. **This is how the open and closed comedones form.**

As I mentioned earlier, closed comedones or whiteheads are more severe because the occlusion of pilosebaceous follicle duct happens more in-depth; therefore, it is impossible to squeeze and "rip" them. Even specific home care takes time to give results.

Going back to the earlier comparison, they are deep located "bombs" which, soon or later, will "explode".

In fact, in clogged follicles, sebum can no longer flow towards the skin surface and accumulates in the lower part of the follicle: this swells and forms a microcyst in the dermis.

Subsequently, as the whitehead increases in size it can become visible and slightly protrude, making the skin rough to the touch.

Let us go back again for a moment and further examine how free fatty acids, which are found in excess in sebum, lead to the formation of free radicals.

For a better understanding of how cosmetics, drugs, and anti-acne dermatological treatments act, it will be important to know the reason why free radicals form (from sebum) and follicular duct wall thickens.

However, the pathogenesis and evolution of acne are very complex processes in which many other factors are involved.

III AND IV FACTOR: INFLAMMATION AND PROLIFERATION OF PROPIONIBACTERIUM ACNES

Further events occur in the occluded follicle:

1. Propionibacterium acnes, a bacterium normally present in the follicular duct, finds the best conditions to live and proliferate (i.e. lower presence of oxygen, greater amount of sebum). And so it begins to multiply.
2. Sebum production does not stop, the accumulation within the blocked follicular duct continues until the wall of the duct itself begins to break down gradually, like a dam collapsing with a river flood.

These events are important to explain the evolution of acne as we will see later.

PAPULAR ACNE AND PUSTULAR ACNE
Why acne is not a skin infection

In the past, acne was treated or considered as a skin infection because a lot of emphasis was put on the growth of bacteria.

There was also fear of contagion, association with disfiguring infectious diseases such as leprosy, and an often unjustified use of antibiotics.

This common way of thinking certainly did not contribute to the welfare of people afflicted by acne (especially if severe) and to the advancement of therapies.

In the past, and sometimes now, antibiotics were seen as the main anti-acne treatment.

They indeed work: there is often an improvement within weeks but this is only an indirect effect – as I will explain later.

Actually, acne is not a skin infection because the bacteria involved normally live on the skin surface and inside of the pilosebaceous follicles.

The 3 most important microorganisms at the skin level are two bacteria: Propionibacterium acnes and staphylococcus epidermidis, and a fungus: malassezia furfur, which is involved in the seborrheic dermatitis manifestation, dandruff and pityriasis versicolor. They normally multiply, but only within certain limits, without creating problems.

Problems arise when the follicular outlet is occluded and the whitehead is formed: Propionibacterium acnes is, in fact, an anaerobic bacterium that lives much better when oxygen is scarce or absent.

Therefore, it finds the ideal conditions for its growth in the closed comedo, taking advantage of it and it multiplies more.

Propionibacterium acnes also produces lipases, which are enzymes that degrade the sebum with further formation of free fatty acids and substances stimulating an immune and inflammatory reaction in the dermis surrounding the whitehead.

These substances are cytokines and chemotactic substances: their function is to start the inflammatory process causing vasodilation (flushing) and the massive arrival of the immune system cells in the area. They are often very small-sized molecules able to cross the space between the cells forming the follicular duct wall, get into the surrounding dermis and recall the white blood cells and other cells related to inflammation. These substances do their work by "attacking" any material or agent recognized as "foreign matter" to the skin tissue.

But this is not the only cause of acne inflammation leading to the formation of **papules and pustules**!

In fact, what is also important is the passage of sebum in the dermis following the partial or total damage of the follicular wall.

Sebum begins to leak into the surrounding dermis through the damaged pilosebaceous follicle wall and is recognised as foreign matter by the immune cells of the dermis (its place is not actually there, but inside the duct and on the skin surface): thus creating an even more intense inflammation.

The skin around the follicle reddens and swells: it forms the red papule or pimple.

The immune system, also activated by the substances produced by propionibacterium acnes, continues to react to the sebum and its molecules: the inflammatory reaction becomes more and more severe and leads to the accumulation of pus.

The pustule forms!

The pus is mostly composed by white blood cells. They liberate substances and enzymes that, like "chemical bombs", aim at destroying microorganisms and foreign substances, but also cause collateral damage: they can harm the dermis until the destruction of small portions of it, thus creating tissue loss and signs of acne scarring.

It is therefore important to understand that when it comes to pustule formation, this may leave a "hole", even a small one. But it will be permanent on the skin!

As we will see later, acne scars can be prevented by minimizing or eliminating the acne inflammation.

So, when is it an actual pimple?

It is a pimple when there is already a visible inflammation and a red papule formed.

The process can either stop here or go ahead with the transformation of the papule into a pustule.

When comedones are accompanied by many papules, the skin condition is called papular acne. When both papules and pustules appear, it is instead called papulopustular acne.

Indeed, one of the acne's characteristics is the simultaneous presence of different lesions, which are at a different evolution stage: in technical terms, it is called evolutionary polymorphism.

In any case, the starting point is always the comedo.

NODULOCYSTIC ACNE

We have covered how papules and pustules form.

But what about those very large pimples which are often called cysts? How do they form?

Those pimples always derive from whiteheads or closed comedones where the inflammatory process is much deeper and located in the heart of the dermis.

Therefore, the size of inflamed tissue is also bigger, in fact, they are **nodules**.

Even the production of pus can be massive: the painful nodule gradually fills with pus, which destroys the overlying dermis and the epidermis. This action sometimes opens up a passage to the surface allowing the pus to spontaneously pour out.

When this type of lesions prevails, we have a clinical picture of **nodulocystic acne**.

It is a severe form of acne for 4 reasons:

- it is deep and often requires treatment via general route
- it is painful: large and deep pimples are very painful
- it is disfiguring during the acute phase
- it is even more disfiguring at a later stage: it is the clinical picture of acne leaving deep and large crater-shaped scars.

Imagine a boy or a girl who sees his/her face transforming in this way: first with big, red, painful, and persistent pimples from which pus and blood comes out. Then, they find large holes on the skin.

From a psychological point of view, is not it devastating?

How can the life of these kids be now and in the future? It is unlikely that there will not be negative impacts on the image of themselves and their self-confidence.

Whether you are personally affected by acne, a parent of a boy/girl suffering from pimples, or just a person who wants to learn more about the subject, it is important to know that any form of acne, (even the initial comedonal stage) can evolve in the nodulocystic type.

When we neglect it or do not take care of it well!

So why wait?

Why not intervene before permanent marks remain?

TEST NO. 1 - FIND OUT WHAT TYPE OF ACNE YOU HAVE

Please read the below text first, then come back up and start the self-examination of your skin.

Look at your face in the mirror.
Can you detect the presence of acne lesions that we have covered so far?

- blackheads
- whiteheads (under the skin)
- red papules (a few mm diameter)
- pustules (red papules with white-yellowish dot full of pus)
- painful nodules (larger and deeper red papules)
- nodulo-cysts (deep nodules full of pus)

Is there only one type of lesion or are there different ones? If yes, which one or which ones?

As previously illustrated, acne is polymorphic: there may be multiple types of lesions at the same time.

Can you see if there is a type of lesion prevailing over the others? Which one?

The prevalence of one or two types of acne lesions characterises the form of acne from which you suffer.

Forms or clinical pictures of acne:

- Comedonal acne
- Comedonal papular acne
- Papular acne
- Papulopustular acne
- Nodular acne
- Nodulocystic acne

Please answer to these questions now:

What is your clinical picture of acne?

Is it inflamed or not?
Is it deep or superficial?

N.B. This test is for guidance only. Diagnosis and treatment of acne and its outcomes are the sole responsibility of your doctor and must necessarily be tailored and adapted to the clinical picture.

THE 4 SECONDARY FACTORS

We have covered the primary factors and how they contribute to the development of acne lesions.

In this chapter, I shall describe other often overlooked factors, which favour the onset of acne, a more severe form of it and the "sabotage" of anti-acne treatments.

They have to do with lifestyle, diet, behaviour and cosmetic habits. Although they are considered as secondary, they help to create (often non-evident) conditions capable of amplifying the effects of the primary factors.

When I talk about my anti-acne method and my personal and specific view on acne treatments, reducing or eliminating the impact of these secondary factors is equally important: with a more global approach, we are going to reduce the "predisposition" to acne.

In short, as you will see, there is a central concept in this book:

acne can be eliminated by undergoing treatments and improving your lifestyle!

It is up to you to follow my advice on how to fight and finally defeat pimples.

COSMETICS

Have you ever noticed:

1.   your acne worsening after Summer?
2.   many whiteheads appearing in a few weeks?
3.   many pimples appearing in a few days?

I bet you have.

It is a very common problem, often so evident and so seemingly inexplicable.

But think about it:

- have you applied sunscreen or suntan oils during Summer?
- have you used a new cosmetic product (cleanser, moisturiser, foundation, etc.) in the last three months?
- have you used a new cosmetic product in the last two weeks?

In the past, cosmetics ingredients included raw materials and other ingredients that were not beneficial for the skin.

Therefore, cosmetic products often triggered allergies, irritations and rashes. At best, they were not pleasant at all as they left the skin shiny and greasy.

In many cases, they also caused the appearance of pimples.

Only in the 70s, more attention was paid to this unexplained and rapid deterioration of acne or to the sudden appearance of acne in women who have never had a single pimple in the past – although having oily skin by nature.

The correlation between the use of cosmetics and the massive appearance of comedones and pimples was studied.

In 1972, the American dermatologist Kligman was the first one to introduce the term "**cosmetic acne**", which indicates the onset or aggravation of acne lesions in patients with apparently normal or acneic skin.

The concept of "**comedogenic power**" of cosmetic products was developed and specific tests were designed to measure it.

However, they noted that a cosmetic product could lead not only to the formation of comedones (whiteheads and blackheads) but, in some cases, also determine the appearance of papules and pustules a few days after its application.

Therefore, a cosmetic product can cause two types of problems:

1. comedogenicity
2. acnegenicity

In the first case, the pilosebaceous follicles are occluded and the comedones form, followed by papules and pustules appearing "in waves"; in the second case, it is a type of chemical irritation causing an acute inflammation of the pilosebaceous follicle, followed by a sudden onset of papules and pustules.

In the first case, the development of comedones is likely to start after a few weeks; in the second case, the appearance of pimples can happen more rapidly, within a few days.

The most frequent problem is that, although some products and some ingredients are not comedogenic, they can have, in some way, "acnegenic power".

A long list of raw materials "responsible" for the formation of comedones was drawn up.

Here is the list so that you can read the ingredients of the cosmetic products that you are probably using.

By the way, in Appendix A, you will find a blog article that will teach you how to read the labels on cosmetic products.

THE MOST COMMON COMEDOGENIC SUBTANCES:

Butyl stearate
Cocoa butter
Corn oil
D&C red dyes
Decyl oleate
Isopropyl isostearate
Isopropyl myristate
Isopropyl neopentanoate
Isopropyl palmitate
Isopropyl stearate
Lanolin acetylated
Linseed oil
Laureth-4

Mineral oil
Myristyl ether propionate

Myristyl lactate
Myristyl myristate
Oleic acid
Oleyl alcohol
Olive oil
Octyl palmitate
Octyl stearate
Peanut oil
Methyl oleate
Petrolatum (vaseline or paraffin)
Safflower oil
Sesame oil
Sodium lauryl sulphate
Stearic acid

I would like to highlight a few in particular:

vaseline, paraffin, mineral oil, lanolin, waxes, unsaturated or free fatty acids, squalene or squalane, castor oil, etc.

A concept that you will often find in this book is that medicine and dermatology are not and cannot be correct sciences because our knowledge of chemistry, molecular biology and skin physiology are not as comprehensive as to mathematically predict the effect of a substance (as well as cures or treatments) on your organism
or skin. Everything is based on statistics and probability.

We are dealing with a biological system, which is alive and interactive!

Furthermore every individual, every skin (and every acne) has its own chemistry and its own way of interacting. Each case is unique!

There are countless factors to consider, some of them are known, others still little known, and some others perhaps unknown: therefore, it is not all black or white, it is not possible to sharply outline this.

The lists and diagrams can help to understand, make predictions or reduce errors, but they are not absolute truth.

In my opinion, this even applies to the comedogenic substances.
Also the American dermatologist Draelos, an authority in the field

of cosmetic dermatology, believes that the problem of comedogenicity is much more complex and cannot be reduced to a simple list. In fact, even products that do not contain the substances listed above, i.e. non-comedogenic, can cause comedonal acne.

It all depends on the individual reaction of each patient against a finished product and not just against a single chemical substance.

In fact, the problem is not actually caused by an individual ingredient, but also by a set of ingredients. Therefore, the formulation and the type of cosmetic product are also important.

For instance, the basic emulsions of creams and lotions can be oil in water (o/w) and water in oil (w/o): with the first emulsion, we obtain products that are less oily, less fat, and (a little...) less moisturising; the second emulsion (w/o) is indicated for very dry skin.

Nowadays, many cosmetic products aimed at young or adult consumers are labelled as "non-comedogenic" and sometimes even "non-acnegenic".

Therefore, in theory, if you have acne and apply one of these products, you should not have any problem, but it is not always the case – unfortunately.

Even cleaning the skin can aggravate acne.

Have you ever noticed a worsening of your skin state and pimples after using a cleanser?

After having washed your face, you feel your skin pulling a little and yet it seems well cleaned and degreased, you do not worry, you even feel a sense of satisfaction: finally, your skin is not greasy and shiny.

You continue to use it, but, in a few days, the skin pulls a little more, maybe it slightly reddens; you think that this is the effect of the purifying power of the cleanser and of its degreasing active ingredients. You will continue... until you see that pimples, instead of drying out and improve, are more inflamed and numerous: an intense worsening occurred.

So, now I want to explain what I have not said before about the importance of **sebum** and **hydrolipidic film**, and their role in the **skin ecosystem**.

We should all know what an ecosystem is: there are concepts and factors such as habitat, species, niche, natural selection, interaction and... balance.

All components interact with each other, none of them are excluded.

Once again, certain bacteria and fungi within the follicles and on the skin surface are stable and harmless "regulars"; they do not cause diseases unless an imbalance occurs and their number suddenly increases or decreases.

In fact, they occupy a "niche" and live in balance with their habitat represented by the skin: if they were not there or if their population were reduced a lot, other bacteria and "pathogens" or "bad" fungi would take over "invading and colonizing" the skin, causing inflammation and disease.

Sebum serves to lubricate, moisturize and protect the skin; therefore, it is not to be seen only as *the culprit* making our skin shiny and full of pimples.

Indeed, it constitutes a large part of the hydrolipidic film, which is also partially formed by sweat, dead cell fragments of the stratum corneum and the natural moisturising factor (NMF).

The hydro-lipid film is a water in oil emulsion (formed by a small part of water in a lot oil or fat represented by sebum), so it is like a very thin layer of rich hydrating lotion covering the skin surface. Normally, under conditions of balance, it has a pH of about 5.5, thus slightly acidic.

This slight degree of acidity has an important protective function: it reduces bacterial and fungal proliferation, keeping the skin free from infections.

And you would ask: what does all this have to do with acne?
Acne is not a bacterial infection, is it?
Of course, bacteria are not very important in acne, but it does not mean that they have no influence: if the skin pH increases the "resident" bacteria, such as Propionibacterium acnes, proliferate more and contribute to worsen the acneic inflammation.

When you use the normal, mild, or Marseille soap, the skin's acidity is compromised; soon after the pimples will become aggravated and the prescribed treatments will not work.

And what about when you buy a special cleanser for oily skin and acne and deterioration equally occur?

As always, distinction has to be made – and this also applies to all anti-acne cosmetic lines. Unfortunately, what they state on product labels and advertising of cosmetics is not 100% accurate.

The classification of the cosmetic product and the claimed effect (in marketing jargon, the so-called "claim") are in fact based on the presence of one or more ingredients that can also have the claimed functional activity. However, the final effect on the skin is determined by the formula as a whole and therefore, also from the rest of the ingredients, such as excipients, surfactants or anything else.

Indeed, if the formulation or the rest of the ingredients are then not really suitable for acneic skin, or do not respect the skin's balance, inserting an active anti-acne ingredient into a product for local use (be it dermocosmetic or medication) is not enough.

For instance, in the case of cleansers: if the cleansing base is formed by aggressive surfactants (with high degreasing power), the hydrolipidic film is largely or even totally removed. Thus, both the acidity of the skin and the epidermal balance will be compromised, the skin will gradually become dry and irritated and the sebaceous glands will react by producing a greater amount of sebum (rebound effect): acne will be likely to deteriorate inexorably.

The skin is an ecosystem: if you "touch" a piece of the puzzle, you can trigger a negative or positive impact on the other pieces and on the whole system.

As our organism, the skin is also dynamically balanced system: it tries to preserve stable conditions to remain normal and healthy.

The secret of general and skin health is in the continuous rebalancing. And the effectiveness of cosmetic products and treatments lies in maintaining the balance conditions and helping to restore them when needed.

That is why the dermatologist's clinical experience and his theoretical and practical knowledge of cosmetology are so important.

The "cosmetic" factor is crucial to the success of acne treatments and therapies.

This factor is an often underestimated component of the therapeutic strategy and, very often, patients are recommended and use products that reduce or eliminate the benefits of the best acne treatments. Among these, surprisingly, there are also those products that are part of specific lines for acne!

As you will see, in my strategic approach to defeat acne, cosmetology is important: the cosmetic habits and the cosmetic products you use are not just an "outline" of the treatment: they are the basis of the therapy itself.

NUTRITION

We are what we eat (sic)
Feuerbach (philosopher)

In the past, people believed that certain foods caused the appearance of pimples. They particularly blamed sweets, chocolate and cold cuts.

Over the years, dermatologists have repeatedly studied the correlation between food and acne, but studies have always given very conflicting results.

However, thanks to the attention brought to the concept of glycemic index of foods, the formation of free radicals (starting from the fats) and the molecular mechanisms of inflammatory processes, other clinical studies were recently carried out on the link between diets rich in refined foods, high glycemic index, and acne severity.

Indeed, acne lesions are more severe (more numerous and more inflamed) for those who consume foods rich in sugars, which suddenly increase a lot the concentration of blood glucose (the sugar found in many foods and that we commonly use to sweeten is the sucrose, which consists of glucose and fructose).

Conversely, if you are on a low glycemic index diet, acne gradually improves!

What happens when we eat foods with high glycemic index?

Blood sugar levels rise rapidly and our pancreas reacts by secreting insulin in the blood, favouring the entry of glucose into cells. In fact, this sugar is key to provide "immediate" power to the cells of our body: for instance, brain cells consume large amounts of oxygen and glucose; if these two elements are missing, our neurons will die quickly!

The insulin increases in the blood in response to a peak of blood glucose, the excess glucose is "pushed" into cells to be used (or stored) and blood sugar returns to normal: thus, the body restores the normal balance conditions which keep it healthy. A reduction (hypoglycemia) or a persistent excess (hyperglycemia) of blood sugar can be harmful, as it happens with diabetes, a disease in which this rebalancing process is not working well.

The problem is that a high glycemic index diet leads to a continuous rise in blood sugar and, consequently, a continuous insulin increase.

This not only makes you fat because insulin pushes glucose into adipose tissue cells where it is stored as fat, but also causes other two important consequences:

1. a persistent hormonal imbalance
2. a persistent increase of insulin in blood and tissues.

The health of our body is based on a dynamic balance: therefore, also the production and the secretion of various hormones in our endocrine system are constantly balanced specifically to maintain the entire system-organism in balance.

Almost every hormone has its antagonist: another hormone with actions and opposite effects.

For example, the insulin lowers glucose in the blood, but glucagon (which is also produced by pancreas) increases it by "pushing or holding it out" of the cells.

This action is also carried out by other hormones, the "stress" hormones, such as cortisol and adrenaline.

In the next chapter, I will talk about stress in more details; I am only mentioning it now because I want you to understand the mechanisms that are set in motion and how everything is connected.

***The body becomes what the foods are, as the spirit
becomes what the thoughts are.***
(Anonymous)

Simple and frequent stressful situations for our body occur when we do not eat for several hours or do sport and blood sugar is reduced. Stress hormones intervene to rebalance the levels and keep the brain and body in perfect working order, enabling you to survive and resist.

Any situation of acute stress, meant in its general sense (e.g. fighting, escaping, a test, a sport competition, anxiety, etc.), leads to an increase in these hormones and a temporary hyperglycemia, useful for the need of "immediate" energy for muscles, brain, and body.

And in case of chronic stress?

There is a continuous secretion of these hormones, cortisol in particular: it is as if we were on a prolonged treatment with cortisone-based drugs. If followed for a long time, we all know that such a cure causes harmful effects on the body and... the skin.

In fact, the onset or worsening of acne is among the many side effects of cortisone-based drugs!

The most immediate effect of a continuous secretion of cortisol (even slightly above normal levels) is to cause a continuous (and mild) hyperglycemia and then a slight and continuous increase of insulin: it is a vicious circle.

And here come the effects of a persistent increase of insulin in blood and tissues.

You must be wondering, does not the insulin rebalance the excess blood sugar? Does it not have a beneficial and stabilising effect?

It has, but an excessive level of insulin (slight yet constant) leads to further imbalances, including, for example, **an increased production of androgens by the ovary** due to the presence of receptors for IGF-1 (insulin-like growth factor) to which insulin is going to bind.

All these imbalances also cause a **reduction of SHBG** (sex hormone binding protein), an important blood protein that binds (and locks) the 80% of circulating male hormones:

when it is reduced, androgens are more "free" to reach the tissues, including the skin. Here the free testosterone is converted into its active form, dihydrotestosterone (DHT).

Everything is connected.

And the troubles caused by the increase of insulin do not stop there. High insulin levels (even with normal blood sugar levels) lead to overweight and obesity, a pathological condition in which there is a greater "resistance" to insulin itself (it does not easily bind to cell receptors). Therefore, it is little used by cells and remains high in the bloodstream and tissues.

A higher concentration of insulin in the blood and intercellular liquids causes an increased production of arachidonic acid, a very important molecule from which eicosanoids derive. These are supposedly "bad" because they have a powerful inflammatory action.

The **eicosanoids** are small molecules present in all tissues, including our skin. Chemically, they are lipoperoxides, oxidised fatty acids.

Always keeping in mind the model of our organism as a continuous balancing system, it is perfectly normal to have the coexistence of "bad" and inflammatory eicosanoids and "good" eicosanoids, with anti-inflammatory and rebalancing action.

The **arachidonic acid**, a precursor of "bad" eicosanoids, forms from the phospholipids of cell membranes.

It is important to note that phospholipids are primarily composed of "essential" polyunsaturated fatty acid (PUFA: the famous omega 3 and omega 6). They are "essential" because our cells cannot "build" them: they can only use those that we introduce with foods.

The PUFAs are also known as vitamin F or AGE **essential fatty acids**.

Basically, they are two: linoleic acid (progenitor of **omega-6**) and alpha-linolenic acid (progenitor of **omega-3**).

The organism is able to produce all other fatty acids precisely from these two molecules,

The arachidonic acid is also formed from linoleic acid (progenitor omega-6) through a chemical reaction called desaturation, favoured by the delta-5-desaturase enzyme.

Indeed, when our diet is too rich in linoleic acid and omega-6 than omega-3, there is an excessive production of arachidonic acid and pro-inflammatory eicosanoids. The result is a state of silent chronic inflammation in our organism.

A diet too rich in refined carbohydrates also leads to the same result because of excessive insulin stimulation.

In fact, insulin activates the delta-5-desaturase, the enzyme which causes its desaturation, the chemical reaction that converts the linoleic acid (omega-6) in arachidonic acid. The enzyme is, instead, inhibited by glucagon (antagonist to insulin) and EPA (eicosapentaenoic acid, omega-3). This explains the anti-inflammatory action of omega 3.

I wanted to explore these biochemical mechanisms in a more technical way ,and the role of the various molecules because they are crucial for understanding the acne inflammation and how it is influenced by nutrition and food supplementation with omega-3 and other substances – these topics will be also covered later in this book.

Anyway, the basic concept is this:

insulin directs the metabolism of omega 6 fatty acids causing an increased production of arachidonic acid and, indirectly, of "bad" eicosanoids in tissues, triggering and then favouring the inflammatory processes in the tissues themselves.

So the **inflammatory state** is powered by:

- persistent excess insulin (for frequent consumption of foods that raise your blood sugar)
- excess of omega-6 fatty acids in your diet
- deficiency of omega-3 fatty acids in your diet
- chronic stress

Inflammation is not always a negative condition: it is one of the main and primitive defence mechanisms of our organism against aggressions.

If the inflammation is persistent and beyond a certain degree, it causes acute or chronic damage: pain, partial death of tissues, degeneration, aging.

Luckily, when balancing mechanisms are efficient, the same cells also produce "good" eicosanoids and other anti-inflammatory substances which mitigate and "turn off" the inflammation, restoring order and balance.

This happens everywhere, even at the level of skin cells.

It is important to remember that essential fatty acids (omega-3 and omega-6) are present in the membrane phospholipids and also in the cells lining the pilosebaceous follicle duct and in the sebum.

Thus, the circle is closed for acne.

Essential fatty acids, necessarily introduced with food because our body is unable to synthesize them, "build" even the skin cell membranes, making them more or less "inflammable" when, respectively, omega-6 or omega-3 prevail.

Moreover, they also enter in the composition of sebum as free fatty acids (polyunsaturated) and, if omega-6 prevail, "bad" eicosanoids are very likely to come from sebum (by oxidation). In this way, we have a state of micro-inflammation at the level of skin surface and follicular duct stimulating hyperkeratosis and follicular occlusion. Thus, both at a general and local level, diet can contribute to the amplification of acne inflammation.

This then explains the link between a pro-inflammatory diet, with high glycemic index foods and unbalanced levels of essential fatty acids, and acne severity.

Therefore, in this case, the popular beliefs were right: in the end, "we are and we become what we eat", and some foods and diet generally have influence on acne.

Later on, in the second part of the book, I will cover this topic again and explain how to adjust and improve your diet in order to reduce the inflammatory state.

STRESS AND EMOTIONS

What is most deep is the skin.
Paul Valéry (writer and poet)

A study carried out by researchers at the University of Oslo (Norway) analysed the health consequences of stress and a diet rich in sugars.

Norwegian researchers highlighted the connection between a "poor diet", which includes sweets, chocolate, and crisps, states of stress affecting adolescents, and the onset of acne.

They also found out that **anxiety and depression worsen acne** or even stimulate its onset in subjects who have never been affected before.

It is probable that this is also due to the so-called **neurogenic inflammation**: the nerve fibres reaching the skin release chemical mediators (neuropeptides) with vasodilator and pro-inflammatory action.

In addition, these states determine a persistent condition of stress, such as a chronic one.

Acne is a skin disease that can represent (either objectively or subjectively) a major blemish. Many studies show that 70% of patients with acne are ashamed, 63% suffer from anxiety, 67% experience a significant reduction in self-esteem and up to 57% of patients reduce their social contacts.

All this feeds negative emotions and represents a condition of "distress", a chronic "bad" stress which is going to further worsen the acne disease itself.

Now, let us see what chain of events is set in motion.

In case of chronic stress, the hypothalamus releases greater quantities of Adrenocorticotropic hormone (ACTH), which stimulates the adrenal glands to produce cortisol (the hormone of chronic stress), and a smaller quantity of male sex hormones such as deipoepiandrosterone (DHEA) and androstenedione (A).

To some extent, does stress stimulate the production of male hormones?

Yes, it does! The activated adrenal glands produce more DHEA and A, which are then converted into testosterone in the liver and skin (sebaceous glands and hair follicles).

Testosterone levels then increase both in the blood and in the skin, where it is then converted into the active form dihydrotestosterone (DHT), which directly stimulates the sebaceous glands.

Thus, the production and secretion of sebum increase and acne appears or worsens!

The hormonal factor, which is represented by male hormones and among the leading causes of acne, is definitely intensified.

However, not only the male hormones increase. Let us see what the increase of cortisol (one of the most powerful hormones produced by our organism) leads to.

Cortisol inhibits the production of "bad" eicosanoids (that is how it carries out its beneficial anti-inflammatory action), but the problem is that it also reduces the formation of "good" eicosanoids – those having a natural anti-inflammatory and rebalancing function.

Furthermore, cortisol increases blood sugar, which causes an increase of insulin. As we know, insulin promotes the release of "bad" eicosanoids that support inflammation and further strengthens the secretion of cortisol.

The end result is a vicious circle that favours a greater production of "bad" eicosanoids, a persistent and comprehensive hormonal imbalance, and a state of mild and chronic inflammation: the so-called silent inflammation.

When acne is associated to chronic stress conditions, it is often very inflamed; pimples are deep and painful.

This is also explained by the "bottom" inflammation caused by the prevalence of "bad" eicosanoids.

Remember when, earlier in this book, I was speaking about cortisol damage in the chapter on nutrition?

We have seen that having an unhealthy diet, with high glycemic index foods, insulin increases, and so does the production of "bad" eicosanoids, starting from essential fatty acids. The secretion of cortisol rises to counter the silent chronic inflammation, but also causing a rise in blood sugar and insulin.

As you may have already learnt, the mechanism triggered by chronic stress has a different starting point at the brain level, but it has the same effects on our bodies and skin.

As the sea level rises with high tide, so does the "high tide" of "bad" eicosanoids and the inflammation of skin and tissue with a wrong diet and chronic, physical, or emotional stress: the pimples appear or worsen!

SMOKING

*Habits begin as cobwebs
and end like chains.*
Spanish proverb

Smoking is a very harmful habit for your body. Like all habits, both good and bad ones, it forms (and strengthens) gradually. It begins in an apparently harmless way, disguised as "moments of relax and leisure" and then it becomes slavery.

Dermatologists have long found that smoking causes premature skin aging, wrinkles, and cutaneous thickening: the skin of smokers and, even more, of female smokers become yellowish and opaque with time.

The harm of nicotine on the skin:

- it produces free radicals in the body, consuming antioxidants useful to the skin such as vitamin C and E
- leads to an accelerated degradation of collagen and elastic fibres and to a thinning of dermis
- causes vasoconstriction with less supply of blood, oxygen, and nutrients to the skin
- causes a minor replacement of epidermal cells and consequently to a thickening of the epidermis (hyperkeratosis)
- alters the composition of sebum and increases its secretion

Precisely because of these effects, smoking stimulates the ductal hyperkeratosis and comedogenesis and can worsen acne scars.

In a British study, the correlation between smoking and gravity of acne scars resulted so strong that researchers confirmed that "the smoke can increase the gravity of the scars in people with acne."

Moreover, smoking can also contribute to the onset of acne during adulthood.

For female adolescent with acne, instead, smoking would increase by 4 times the possibility to suffer from acne even in adulthood.

In another study, published in 2007 in the British Journal of Dermatology, researchers at the San Gallicano of Rome observed 1,000 women in the age range of 25-50 and described a particular type of non-inflammatory acne, characterised by many microcysts and comedones spread evenly all over the face, especially on the cheeks and forehead: post adolescent comedogenic acne (CPAA).

This form of acne was found to be not only the most common form of acne among the participants of the study, but also the type of acne that affected smokers the most.

Therefore, the results of various studies suggest that you should avoid smoking, if you want to keep your skin clean and free from pimples or if you do not want acne to worsen.

TEST NO. 2 - FINDING YOUR WAY WITH TREATMENTS

If you have not already done it, **please complete test no. 1 first -** *Find out what form of acne you have*

What form of acne do you have?

- Comedonal acne
- Comedonal papular acne
- Papular acne
- Papulopustular acne
- Nodular acne
- Nodulocystic acne

Then answer these groups of questions with yes or no:

Have you only treated acne with cosmetics so far?
If yes, did you get benefits from it?

If you answered yes to both questions: you have a quite mild acne but there is room for further improvement.

If you answered yes to the first question and no to the second: you probably have a form of acne requiring treatment with local or general medication.

Have you already followed an anti-acne treatment involving drugs in the past?
If yes, did you get benefits from it?

If you answered yes to both questions: you have a form of acne that is responding well to treatment and can definitely improve.

If you answered yes to the first question and no to the second: your form of acne tends to resist treatment with drugs, therefore, it might be necessary to take general medication or stronger drugs.
It is also possible that the drugs were not suitable to your form of acne.

Have you already followed long therapies involving general medication?
Have you ever followed a therapy taking isotretinoin orally?
Did you get benefits from it?

If you answered yes to all questions: your form of acne, although serious, responds well and can still improve.

If you answered yes to the first two questions and no to the third: it is a severe form of acne and possibly resistant to treatment.
Perhaps you only need to change the treatment and pay special attention to cosmetics you use; outpatient treatments might be also necessary.

N.B. This test is for guidance only. Diagnosis and treatment of acne and its outcomes are the sole responsibility of your doctor and must necessarily be tailored and adapted to the clinical picture.

WHY STILL WAIT?

The person who waits for a long time
can always wait a little longer
Gabriel García Márquez (writer)

If you suffer from acne, you know very well that the waves of pimples come and go, and there are times when you may experience a sudden worsening for several factors.

It is precisely in these moments that pimples increase in number and become more painful and deep, and acne leaves its marks on your face – they are scars that will hardly disappear; in the best case scenario, they can improve.

So why wait that pimples leave marks and scars?
Is not it much easier to prevent it with an appropriate anti-acne treatment?

Once again, it all depends on you, on your decisions and your determination.

Waiting for your acne to improve or disappear on its own is useless, counterproductive, and harmful: unfortunately, that is unlikely to happen.

It is much better to start treatments and applying the anti-acne method as soon as possible!

The earlier you start, the better: we are approaching the first step.

You will see that the path I will suggest you take is not as complex as you might think, it is doable and you can do it.

You only need to follow phases, build habits and a routine that will finally lead you to the desired result.

In the second part of the book, we will see the pillars on which we will found our war on pimples.

NOTE:

PART II

CURE ACNE IN 7 STEPS

A journey of a thousand miles begins with a single step
Lao Tze (philosopher)

We covered the primary and secondary causes of acne and how pimples form because it is important to understand all the mechanisms at the basis of the problem before you tackle it.

Now it is time to start our journey through the 7 basic steps that will lead us to achieve our goal: fight pimples and win against acne.

As you will see, these 7 steps are in sequence, which needs to be followed as it is presented because each step strengthens the next.

If you want, you can imagine it as a staircase or a pyramid: each step takes you to the summit.

There are no shortcuts.

1. **Motivation and Objectives**
2. **Self-esteem and stress control**
3. **The dermatologist**
4. **Care and dermatological treatments**
5. **Avoid the mistakes that worsen pimples**
6. **The anti-acne diet**
7. **Winning in style**

The first two steps concern you in particular: you need to prepare yourself to face acne treatments with the right mental attitude.

This will give you the strength to begin, endure, and persevere. The third and the fourth steps are the heart of the anti-acne strategy: I will explain how to choose the dermatologist who will follow you, I will discuss the pros and cons of care and dermatological treatments to fight acne, and my concept of the four pillars of an effective anti-acne treatment.

In the fifth step, you will discover the 12 mistakes to avoid while treating pimples and that might make any cure ineffective.

The sixth and seventh step relate to your lifestyle, from eating habits to your daily routine, how to change certain habits for the better to help improve acne and have better skin and a face free from pimples.

STEP I: REASONS AND OBJECTIVES

Energy and persistence conquer all things.
Benjamin Franklin (inventor)

The first step is the beginning of everything: it mainly concerns the necessary motivation to start treating acne.

As a dermatologist, I have seen many patients suffering from acne but had never taken the decision to get rid of it with determination and commitment.

Right, when you are an adolescent and young, you might feel existential discomfort and disorientation; you are in a moment where your image and identity change. In fact, there may be other priorities: being accepted by your peers, your opposite sex, and parents with whom you come into conflict.

However, this cannot and should not justify the lack of self-care, also because the top priority is, indeed, accepting yourself and the changes occurring in your body during adolescence.

And I do not think I exaggerate when I say that dedication to fighting pimples can also be a way to help strengthen personality and self-esteem, it can be really useful to your personal growth.

Indeed, finding determination within yourself, setting a goal, and committing with patience, perseverance, and method are fundamental virtues for success, not only against (the hated) pimples but also in many other situations in life.

Therefore, it may represent a real educational experience!

Please read and see PART II as the beginning of a journey that will give you strength, a lot of practical advice and a way to finally defeat acne.

The first step is to make the decision to finally win against pimples, but, as you will see, in order to make a decision you should have:

- information and belief that do not hinder or disorient you
- the ability to set goals
- a strong motivation to act.

The following pages will seem a little strange, maybe off topic, because they are going to tackle these issues specifically. Please bear in mind that it is not digressions, banality or loss of time.

The concepts and exercises that you will encounter are crucial:

they will help you to clear your head, see yourself and acne in a different way, remain strong, change negative attitudes, respect and value yourself more.

WHAT PREVENTS YOU TO FIGHT PIMPLES EFFECTIVELY

It is easier to break an atom than a prejudice.
Albert Einstein (physicist)

It is true that motivation may often fail for various reasons, but there are also ways of thinking and common beliefs that are able place limits on our determination.

They are what I call the false myths on acne.

REALISATION

Every day, you look at your face in the mirror and notice the presence of a few or many (or even too many) pimples and you say yourself that, one day, sooner or later, you will begin a treatment: a war against acne to have a cleaner face and recover your beauty.

You are well aware of how pimples "ruin" your face and how this makes you suffer when you are around friends who may have clearer skin and look better.

Once again, you promise yourself that one day, sooner or later, you will begin a treatment, even if you do not know exactly which.

You read on forums, or heard from friends and relatives, about some people who tried certain products or treatments and obtained successful results. But also about others who tried everything without seeing any improvement and are consequently desperate or resigned.

You also alternate days when you would like to face the problem and days of resignation and inertia.

There is only a reason behind the fact that you have borne the pimples (and all their negative psychological consequences) on your face so far: you have not really made the firm decision to fight acne.

Making a decision
Deciding does not mean hope and wait, but implementing a behaviour and moving towards a goal.

Making a decision and acting is an act of will and responsibility based on information and belief.

Start your challenge by asking yourself some questions:

__What prevents you from taking action?__
__What prevents you from starting to fight pimples?__

You might already have all necessary information and read everything you need to know about acne, but you will never be able to eliminate or keep pimples under control, if you do not start acting.

It is also true that what motivates us in our decisions and actions are determined beliefs (and information) which can stimulate or block us.

Beliefs are made of thoughts and opinions (heard by parents, relatives, or friends) that later became "metropolitan legends" and myths accepted and recognised as truth by almost everyone. They can be totally false, totally true or partially true i.e. inaccurate, but always influence attitudes and behaviours.

There are also widespread opinions that have certainly a scientific basis but if misinterpreted, they can lead to wrong conclusions and consequently to ineffective behaviours: they disorient us and lead us completely astray!

I have identified six "myths" that often come out during examinations and talks with patients and that might lead you to believe that fighting pimples is useless or does not entirely depends on you:

Acne depends on age, *so it is destined to heal on its own over time*

Acne depends on family history, *so you cannot do anything about it and you have to get over it*

Acne is a normal condition: almost everyone has pimples, *so it is not a disease and trying to treat it is useless.*

Acne depends on food intolerance or poor diet, *so you only need to identify and avoid harmful foods and it will heal*

Acne will heal only when you have found *the right treatment or dermatologist*

There are treatments and remedies to quickly and permanently defeat acne, *so you only need to find them and, in a* *few days and effortlessly, you will finally be healed forever.*

We will now debunk these myths one by one; again, they are not 100% wrong as they have some truth, but, in any case, they represent beliefs and assumptions that lead us to indecision or to take incorrect decisions about which path to follow to effectively treat pimples.

Acne depends on age, *so it is destined to heal on its own over time*

It is true that acne can make its appearance in adolescence because of the male hormones produced in both men and women.

It is also true that in mild cases pimples crumble and disappear after 20-25 years of age, perhaps without leaving any signs.

However, it is often true and frequent that:

- acne lasts many years, even in adulthood
- if they are not treated, pimples tend to worsen
- pimples can leave spots and, in particular, permanent scars
- the persistence of pimples in the adolescent or young adult leads to psychological distress with a negative impact on self-esteem and therefore on social life and sexual relationships

Acne depends on family history, *so you cannot do anything about it and you have to get over it*

True. As in many diseases, also in acne there is a given familiar and hereditary predisposition, and this is a truth to be accepted with serenity.

But accepting does not mean having to resign.

If parents had acne, it is likely that their children will have it too. However, the predisposition and severity of acne can vary from individual to individual.

It is not an inevitable fate to which you should resign yourself to: you can treat acne and keep it under control and, above all, you can avoid the possibility that it worsens or becomes severe.

Acne is a normal condition: almost everyone has pimples, *so it is not a disease and trying to treat it is useless.*

It is not quite correct to think that acne is normal just because it is very common.

It is a real skin condition that manifests with various levels of severity: it is better and useful to treat it even during its early stages.

In good faith and with all the best intentions, parents often used this myth in an attempt to reassure their children because they perceive the psychological and emotional discomfort. But, unfortunately, these statements do not take into account a fact that will soon become evident to their children:

Individual pimples will go away within a few days or weeks but acne lasts for years.

In any case, if the parents did not take care of it and they were lucky because they have suffered from a mild acne, this is not a good reason not to encourage their children to treat it properly.

Acne depends on food intolerance or poor diet, *so you only need to identify and avoid harmful foods and it will heal*

It is true that nutrition may be important in the manifestation of acne and its degree of inflammation, but it is also true that it is a secondary factor and does not replace the dermocosmetic and dermatological treatments.

Avoiding certain foods can help improve acne, but it is not true that it will only heal with a special diet.

Acne will heal only when you have found *the "right" treatment or dermatologist*

True. For all forms of acne, there is the "right" and appropriate therapy: the one which gives you a clear and visible improvement.

But it is also true that each person, each skin, and each disease or form of acne reacts differently – even to the same treatment. We cannot generalise and there is not a valid standard treatment for everyone.

Unfortunately, medicine and dermatology are not exact sciences!

No illusions, a therapy has always been considered an "attempt" to improve (or treat) the disease: according to his experience and his talent, the dermatologist can more or less "predict" the

benefits, but you still need to "try" the therapy in order to see the real effects it has on your skin and on your pimples.

It is true that the initially prescribed treatment may not be the "right" one or not be giving you the desired improvements.

But it is also true that the anti-acne treatments take time to give results and your skin needs time to rebalance itself, helped by therapies.

It is also true that you cannot desperately chase the "right" treatment in the hope of finally setting yourself free from acne. Actually, the true "right" treatment is the one that will gradually let you keep acne under control: from the disappearance of inflamed pimples to a cleaner skin, with a significant reduction of whiteheads, blackheads and new pimples.

It is true that the dermatologist may be the "right one", if he devotes much of its work to treat acne, if he has a good knowledge of cosmetology, if he does not underestimate the aesthetic side of skin diseases and if he really listens to you.

But it is also true that there is not doctor or dermatologist able to finally heal your acne in a few days: be wary of those who promise you rapid and definitive miracles.

Looking for the "right" treatment or dermatologist might turn out to be an endless research for its own sake: an excuse to delay the start of any treatments.

There are treatments and remedies to quickly and permanently defeat acne, *so you only need to find them and, in a few days and effortlessly, you will finally be healed forever.*

True. There are treatments that allow a rapid disappearance (or within a reasonable time) of pimples and comedones (I have written a lot about the benefits of chemical peel), but it is equally true that rapid improvement does not mean ultimate healing from acne: it is just an important first step for home acne treatments to be more effective.

Individual pimples will go away within a few days or weeks but acne lasts for years.
Your skin will always remain prone to acne, so constant (but not necessarily binding) and drug-based treatments will be necessary.

True. The anti-acne treatments cost time and money, but when they are very expensive and pledge definitive healing, you should seriously doubt their advertised and boasted effectiveness.

The truly most effective acne treatments are the most simple; they do not complicate life, but they do require commitment, method and perseverance.
You can now decide yourself whether you want begin fighting pimples by doing everything you need to do or still believe in these myths that lead you to be passive, resign or treat your acne in an ineffective way.

DECISIONS AND OBJECTIVES
HOW TO START WINNING AGAINST ACNE

How do you eat an elephant?
One bite at a time!
African proverb

As previously explained, I am sure that you can win against pimples: it is a battle that you can win, but you have to fight.

YOU are the only person that must fight.

This 7 steps path is, in fact, only the beginning of the anti-acne treatment and it includes the necessary steps for skin care and your war against pimples to become your daily routine.

The purpose of this path is to give you a method, creating new habits and a healthy lifestyle for your skin and not only.

It is a beginning: this does not mean that you will not see benefits during the first weeks.

When a missile is launched into space, the majority of engine power and fuel is used to detach from the ground and overcome the force of gravity. As the missile takes off, it will need less power: the flight and the maintenance of the route become increasingly less challenging.

And so it will be with acne: the beginning is much more difficult and often boring: it will require more energy and commitment.

Once you have the command of your routine of anti-acne treatments, you will begin to see improvements and everything will become easier, simpler, more satisfying.

Are you sure you really have decided to treat the pimples?

Making a decision does not mean hope and wait, but implementing a behaviour and moving towards a goal.

Why do not you start taking care of your skin today?

If you reflect for a moment, you can easily realise that, deep down inside of you, even doing nothing to fight pimples is a decision! Yes, until now, you have probably just decided not to fight acne! Maybe you have been thinking about it for months, you can no longer stand the pimples disfiguring your face, you just want them all to disappear. But, in the end, you decided not to do anything or to do some attempts without belief and give up after a few days or weeks. Starting the war against acne only depends on you and your decisions.

Perhaps because of this book, you might have now become an expert connoisseur of acne, its causes, its treatments, but then if you do not really decide to begin treating pimples, you will never be able to win against acne.

And to begin means taking action.
The action is not made of words, but of behaviour!
You could say you have decided that tomorrow or next week you will take an appointment for a dermatological examination and begin the treatment for pimples, but if you do not do it now, it means that you have not made a real decision yet.

Of course, the decision can be only yours and **must be linked to the action**; the action is made of behaviours, and a set of consistent behaviours become habits, routines, and then lifestyle.

LIFESTYLE

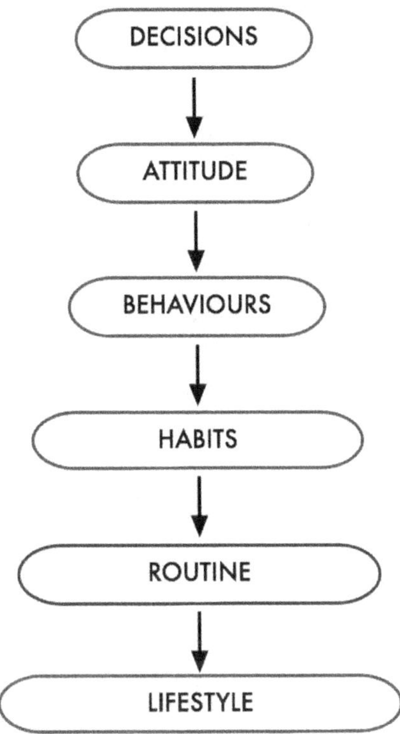

For an effective action, we need to set **goals**, acquire or enhance our skills, and utilise **adequate tools or means**.

Let us talk about these concepts further.
It will be useful later...

What are the goals?

There may be different levels of goals: intermediate and final goals. In our case, we can set a **main or ultimate goal (purpose or goal)**: to win acne. And in order to achieve it, we need to follow a path with various **intermediate goals**, i.e. the many steps that will lead us to the final achievement.

However, goals are not hopes or aspirations.

You could even scream to the entire world, with all the force and despair that you have, "I want to win against acne! I want a clean skin without pimples!" and then do nothing or make some short-term attempts.

Or **you can set deadlines** with intermediate goals, like stages to complete before the ultimate goal.

A goal without a deadline is just a simple desire, a vain hope.

Setting and meeting the deadline is what makes you act: here is why you need a plan or a path to follow in order to fight pimples.

That is why you will need to learn how to set goals: a fundamental skill that will be useful in many areas and also for the future.

What are the skills?

If you think about it, you already have many skills, maybe you play a musical instrument, you know how to use a particular software, you know how to perfectly set up your phone or tablet, you can draw, you know how to play football, etc.

Having a skill means knowing how to do something in specific, with greater or lesser mastery.

For instance, if you are a computer or Internet whiz, it is very likely that you have been spending a long time, or even whole nights, on it.

As you will see, there are also some fundamental and useful skills to learn to win against acne.

What are the means?

Means are tools, skills and methods through which we can achieve our goals.

With its 7 steps path, this book is a means, just a simple tool at your disposal useful to achieve the goal of set yourself free from pimples.

METHOD

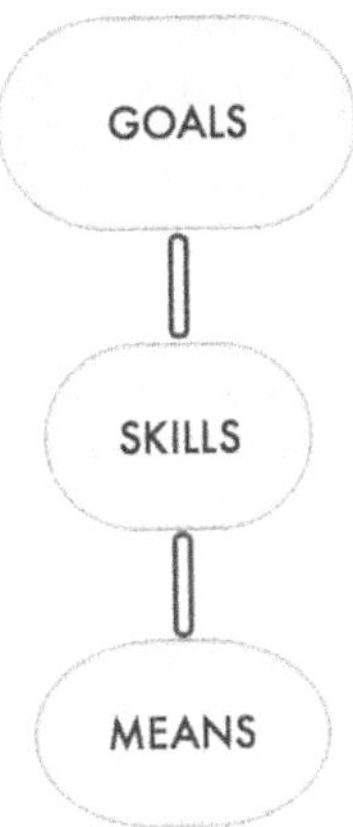

How to set and achieve goals

We have already covered what goals are and how to distinguish the real ones from the fake ones:

the real goals have deadlines and are related to action.

How do we set goals?
Imagining, deciding, and planning.
Imagining how and what we will get when we achieve a given goal.
With the following exercise, you will train your ability to imagine that you can set yourself free from pimples. As you will repeat it several times each day, you will strengthen your will to take action.

EXERCISE NO. 1: one step away from the action

Take at least 20 minutes to isolate yourself and relax, and to calmly reflect:

Can you imagine your skin more and more free from pimples and blackheads?

Think how, day after day, and week after week, your skin purifies thanks to the care you follow with perseverance and determination: imagine how pimples, blackheads and whiteheads gradually decrease on your face and on your skin, until they disappear completely and finally leave a beautiful, bright, clean, and smooth face.

While you see this gradual improvement, you can inevitably realise that it is a goal and a result that can be achieved: so many other people like you have been through this and they succeeded, perhaps starting with a even more serious situation.

How to we achieve goals?

Deciding planning with precise timing, identifying and developing the skills and the means we need to achieve them effectively.

With this 7 steps path I am actually already suggesting a plan with intermediate goals.

Consider it an initial push to exercise your willpower to meet deadlines and to achieve the final goal: controlling acne and maintaining skin as healthy and beautiful as possible.

Now you have your plan of action!

You will decide times and deadlines, though. You are the only one that can decide this... Even depending on speed with which you read this book and your motivation. Right, reading is definitely not enough; step by step, you will need to do what you read, do both tests and exercises.

Therefore, I suggest you set a first tight deadline: in four weeks, you read and re-read the book and begin to apply the 7 steps.

The time taken to achieve the goal only depends on you!

You only need to be a little organised to avoid excuses such as "I did not have time to read", "I have no time to do the exercises", "I do not have time right now", "Unfortunately, I have other more important things to do", "I do not have time to apply the lotion or wash my face."

There are no excuses: the world's best method will not replace your will and your action!

In fact, it is up to you to put this method into practice every day, because only with determination and perseverance you will see the benefits.

In order to obtain a result, and to achieve any goal in life, not only means and skills are important: the fundamental secret is having a great will!

Time management: how to find time

In order to find the time to read this book, apply the method, do the treatment, from washing your face to remove make-up and apply lotions, you will need to commit and act, avoiding less important activities although enjoyable as watching television, listening to music or sleeping.

It is actually about truly dedicating a few minutes to all that every day, but so far, perhaps, you have never done it.

Why?

If you think about it, one of the most generic but frequent apologies is "I did not have time".

Apparently, it all makes sense: you had other commitments (from studying to working, from friends to having fun) and you can brilliantly justify the fact that you have not yet started to treat acne or follow the recommended therapy.

Some excuses or strategies for postponing or avoiding to start treatment:

- I have no time…
- I will start tomorrow …
- I am tired now…
- I have to study now…
- I am already late…
- I will start when I am ready…

- I am not in the mood...
- I am waiting for an improvement...
- I am looking for the right treatment...
- I am looking for the right dermatologist...
- It is a hereditary problem, I cannot help it...

How can you avoid the excuses?

First, you need to decide to fight acne then develop the **ability to manage your time**... or rather the **ability to manage yourself!**

You will see that this will be also very useful for many other occasions in the future: it is one of the most important abilities, perhaps the most important – it will allow you to master your life.

It is a skill that you already have and that, somehow, you already use when you organise your homework doing, prepare for school assignments, or even to find the time to have fun with friends.

METHOD

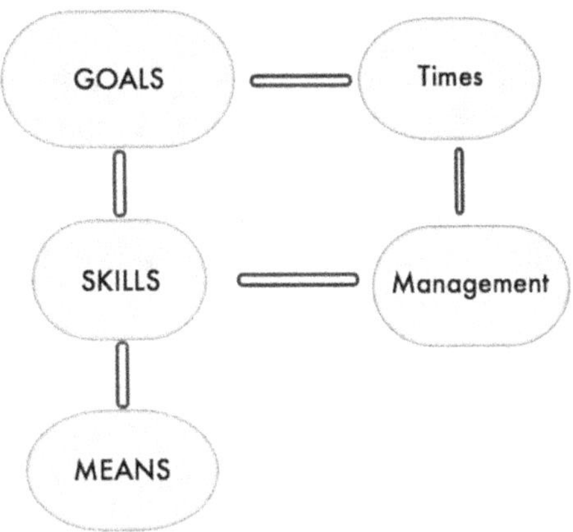

At the base of effective self-management there is the distinction between two concepts: **importance and urgency**. Only in this way, we are able to determine what our priorities are according to the goals that we set out to achieve.

You will then have to learn to distinguish between important and urgent actions.

It all depends on the goals you set!

In fact, only commitments and really important actions have to do with the achievement of your goals.

The rest are urgent commitments or actions of little importance and therefore unnecessary.

Those that are urgent are dictated precisely by urgencies, which are often external pressures that concern the achievement of goals of other people (friends, relatives, etc.) instead of yours.

Sometimes even urgent ones may still be important and therefore they must necessarily and quickly be done to make room for more important things, although less urgent.

How important is for you to have a face with no pimples?

Is it also urgent?
Really?
Are you sure? Is it really your goal?

If you purchased this book, you are reading it and want to apply its suggestions, so I take for granted that eliminating pimples is important (and urgent) for you – this is your goal.

But do not delude yourself: reading this book or having a dermatological examination will not lead to results if you do not follow the advice and apply the prescribed treatments.

You will necessarily need to find the time for the treatments.

Think of what other excuses you have found so far for not doing so and for postponing it every time...

Let us go back to the previous concepts and put them into practice.

The purpose or ultimate goal is to achieve a visible improvement of the skin to increase self-esteem and motivation, thus creating a virtuous circle:

progressive improvement - motivation - continuation of treatments - improvement

reversing the cycle and then defeating the vicious circle:

worsening - demotivation - quitting the treatments - progressive worsening.

I want this to be clear: the 7 steps path does not replace the dermatologist and dermatological treatments, but it rather includes them.

Furthermore, the anti-acne treatment does not end with the 7 steps **(intermediate goals)** and with the times you have chosen because the ultimate goal is to build and follow a method that goes from skin care to food and lifestyle: a set of treatments and healthy habits to be constantly applied.

Every single step is not to be considered standing on its own because they are all connected: each step strengthens the next and all the others at the same time.

So, this is not a linear path from point 1 to point 7 but a circular one: while initially it will be appropriate to follow them in order, at a later time feel free to retrace previous steps to read them again and re-apply its principles and exercises. Actually, it will be necessary and useful.

The fundamental **skills** to develop or improve in this first step:

- how to set and achieve goals
- how to manage time and yourself
- how to improve your mood and motivation.

The **intermediate goals** are:

- Increasing motivation and determination to treat your skin
- Setting and achieving the goal: managing yourself
- Creating positive moods and increasing motivation

They are **small and simple commitments**, even apparently unrelated to each other, but they will all gradually change your habits, making you quit behaviours harmful for your skin.

There will be some more with the next step to come, until you build a daily routine and a healthier lifestyle for your skin.

INCREASING MOTIVATION AND DETERMINATION TO TREAT YOUR SKIN

Sow a thought and reap an action, sow an action and reap a habit, sow a habit and reap a character, sow a character and reap a destiny.
Anonymous

In order to achieve this goal (as any other goal in life) you first have to practice to develop and improve will and motivation.

They are the pillars that support your decision to fight pimples and are the fuel to trigger action.

EXERCISE NO. 2: everything is possible

Take at least 20 minutes to isolate yourself and relax, and to calmly reflect:

Think of your older brothers and sisters, or even friends or friends older than you: perhaps, many of them have suffered from acne, some of them did not follow treatments, others treated it inadequately or ineffectively, others managed to fight pimples and they now have a better and a cleaner skin.

Reflect on the fact that acne is just a temporary imbalance condition. Think how your skin can regain its balance and its beauty only if you help it with treatments.

There are several effective treatments: winning against acne is also possible for you now.

EXERCISE NO. 3: This is not a dream

Take at least 20 minutes to isolate yourself and relax, and to calmly reflect:

Look at your face in the mirror, see how many and what kind of pimples there are now.

Think about how pimples limit your relationships with friends or in your daily activities at school, university, gym, etc. Think of any situation where you feel embarrassed or rejected.

Also remember your feelings and the words that you say to yourself in those moments. Reflect upon this, I bet they are not encouraging at all, are they?

Spend two minutes breathing slowly and deeply. Now, try not to think about anything and just focus on your breathing.

Now imagine your skin smooth and clean or remember how it was when you did not have acne and how you were happy and peaceful, how you were feeling good and how you could feel the same way if you eliminated pimples.
Reflect upon how your feelings, behaviours, mood, and life could be positive if your face had no pimples, if you did not suffer from acne.
It would be a completely different life, right? This is not a dream, but it is goal that you can achieve.

Repeat these exercises every day for at least a week, and every time you want or you feel the need to.
They will progressively strengthen your will to act, even though you may not realise that right away.

How to create positive moods and increase motivation

We are what we think. All that we are arises with our thoughts. With our thoughts, we create our world.
Buddha

What are moods?

They are emotional states, made of thoughts and feelings.
Thoughts are made up of images, words and sounds that we remember or we build with our mind, accompanied by feelings and physical reactions that correspond to emotions.

Thoughts and emotions are usually temporary (they can last seconds or minutes): they come and go like clouds in the sky, while moods are more persistent than thoughts and emotions: they can become habitual and therefore more durable (hours, days, weeks, and months).

We may have moods of joy, serenity, confidence, hope, and states of mind of sadness, anger, frustration, despair: so, both positive and negative.

You already know that positive emotions and moods make us feel good and support us in our actions, they give us strength and
energy while the negative ones have the opposite effect, they weaken us and block us.

It is important to understand that moods do not happen by chance. We are the ones who constantly create them and we can hone this ability to build better and positive ones, which are useful to us and able to make us feel good.

Indeed, as we create them, we can also change them.

How do we create emotions and moods?

As previously stated, the building blocks of emotional states are thoughts and feelings.

Thoughts, in particular, are made of images, sounds and words. Thinking is an incessant activity: we constantly build or recall images, feel or remember sounds, smells and tastes, we talk to ourselves.

It is like we constantly projected films in our mind.

Do not you think it is better to project positive films? Those that make you feel good and that help and support the achievement of your goals?

The quality of our thoughts and the resulting emotions and moods depends on the quality of the images, sounds, smells and tastes, and the words we say to ourselves.

What most negatively affects the mood of the patient with acne is looking himself/herself in the mirror and say humiliating and depressing words:

"I look horrible"
"I am scary and disgusting"
"I have a disfigured face full of pimples"
"No one will ever like me"
Therefore, in the inner dialogue with yourself, you make assessments and express negative judgments about your appearance and the possibility to treat and win against acne.

And this brings you to experience negative feelings and emotions such as frustration, anxiety, and depression.

The inner dialogue is ongoing and if these thoughts are frequent, you are unconsciously doing a real brainwashing: you get used to feeling upset and to self-loathing and start to convince yourself that there is nothing you can do to improve.

Words form the thread on which we string our experiences.
A. Huxley (Writer)

EXERCISE NO. 4: Observe and transform the inner dialogue

The words you say are your thoughts. The way you say them to yourself (the tone of your voice) corresponds to the way you think.

We are so used to speaking to ourselves and to keeping ourselves company...
We always tell ourselves about judgments and evaluations on the various situations we encounter people, objects, and also ourselves.

It is a normal and natural process and, in most cases, it takes place unconsciously.
It is important to become aware of the thoughts that constantly run through your mind.
You need to develop the ability to pay attention to your thoughts.

In particular, train yourself to become aware of your thoughts about pimples.

Answer these questions and think:

What words do you say to yourself?
Are these words encouraging or depressing?
Are these words of affection or despise?

What tone of voice do you use when you address yourself or express judgments on yourself?
Is it calm and gentle or respectful?
Is it contemptuous or angry?
Is it melancholic and whiny?

Is it desperate?

In what circumstance do you have negative words for yourself? Before dealing with others?
When you are among others?
When other people make positive or negative appreciation about you? When you are alone?
When you are in front of the mirror?

Become conscious of all these moments.

The jokes and the opinions of others

Unfortunately, these evaluations are often reinforced (and validated) by jokes and similar opinions expressed by others: friends, strangers, relatives and parents too.
Sometimes adolescents can be cruel and aggressive towards their peers, often without even realising it.

How can you defend yourself against jokes and opinions of others?

What really matters is not the words that they say to you but *how you react to these words*: you can feel despair, become angry or depressed, or choose to react by turning them into a stimulus to start to heal or continue treatments with even more determination!

Yes, if you want, you can transform anger and frustration into greater determination!

EXERCISE NO. 5: How to create a shield to the opinions of others

- Review, as a film, a situation where others joked or more or less explicitly said negative words about the appearance of your face and pimples.

- Think and become aware of the emotional reaction you had when hearing those words. What hurt you the most: the words of others or the words you said to yourself (e.g. they are right) in that moment?

- Turn yourself off for a moment, think of something else for a few seconds.

- Go back to that situation, but now look at it as if you were a spectator: look at yourself in the middle of the scene and those who say those words.

- Once again, look at it again, always as if you were a spectator, you hear the other person saying those words changing the quality of voice: lowering the volume or reducing the speed, as if you were hearing it in slow motion, or increasing it to deform it and make it ridiculous.

What feelings and emotions are you feeling when you look at the situation in this way? Do not you think that they are less intense or even different?

Repeat points 4 and 5 of this exercise, carrying on experimenting and having fun by changing the film in the most bizarre ways: you can change your appearance by making yourself taller and bigger than the other person, or making him/her smaller until he/she becomes a talking dot or turning him/her into a small animal, a gnat or an amorphous and harmless object.

You will definitely laugh about it at some point...

Every time you find yourself in a similar situation, think that you can change it on the spot, as if you were taking and transforming the scene from the outside.

EXERCISE NO. 6: How to turn frustration into determination

If you are frustrated because you suffer from acne and pimples do not improve this is a good sign!
I am not joking. Think about it and you will realise that frustration is an emotion of anger for a goal you are not able to achieve, therefore it means that defeating the acne is a goal you are imposing on yourself, perhaps you only need a method to achieve it.

Or it is probably more due to too high or unrealistic expectations: you expect that pimples disappear within one or a few weeks and that they will not appear anymore. Unfortunately, it does not work like this, you cannot delude yourself, look for the right treatment or remedy that works wonders.

You will just end up feeling disappointed and frustrated, and perhaps you would quit or change treatments or dermatologist before you see the benefits.

From what you have read in this chapter, you will have certainly learnt that what you think and your attitude are important.

In order to fight pimples effectively, we always need to rely on these three factors:

1. your attitude
2. treatment
3. dermatologist

The frustration is a sign that the goal has not been achieved yet or is moving away. If you want to achieve your goal, you need to change strategy, but, as you will see later, you need to think carefully about which of the three factors you need to act upon.

Remember: no obstacle is insurmountable, you can win against acne!

Every step you take, every improvement you will see on your skin (thanks to your efforts) will bring you a feeling of satisfaction and relaxation: your brain will release a small amount of endorphins, a natural drug called the hormone of wellness. The brain rewards you every time you achieve a goal that you set, though small, thus reinforcing your self-discipline.

However, the opposite is also true: when we cannot achieve a goal or we do not we keep the commitments with ourselves, we

feel frustrated, our self-esteem reduces and anxiety and stress increase.

These will be the topics of the next chapter.

STEP II: IMPROVING THE PERCEPTION OF YOURSELF AND MANAGING STRESS

And we are at the second step. In the first step, we debunked the myths and false legends which blocked or limited the effectiveness of your initiative in treating pimples, you learnt how important it is to take a real decision, the power to set goals and to respect given deadlines, manage your time and commitments of your daily life according to the criteria of urgency and importance.

Finally, we saw some exercises to increase motivation and determination: real action fuels.

We go on to the next level now: it is necessary to increase self-confidence to further strengthen the will to succeed and begin to free ourselves from mental (and physical) toxins of stress, anxiety, and pessimism.

The fundamental **skills** to develop or improve in this second step are:

- how to improve self-perception
- how to keep stress under control

In order to achieve the intermediate goals:

- increase self-esteem
- reduce emotional stress

We have already covered how it may be useful to handle stress, also caused by acne itself, and improve mood in general: if we act
on these factors, we act on the psycho-neuro-immune-endocrine system, thus reducing the overall inflammatory potential.

Both your body and your skin will benefit from it: the intensity of acne inflammation will attenuate.

HOW TO INCREASE YOUR SELF-ESTEEM

The man who considers his life as devoid of sense is not only unhappy but also incapable of living.
Albert Einstein (physicist)

What is self-esteem?
Self-esteem is the perception of your value as a person and of your qualities and skills.

Like all perceptions, it is only a subjective evaluation, a way to interpret and see yourself, so it is not necessarily accurate or correct.

Anyway, this vision has a considerable impact on our attitudes, our behaviours and, ultimately, our lives. A low self-esteem can lead to a vicious circle, with ever-worsening attitudes and moods:

- Excessive need for approval
- Lack of trust in our own abilities
- Pessimism and feeling of helplessness
- Victimhood
- Depression

And certainly, none of this will help us to achieve the goal of winning against acne.

The good news is that the cycle can be reversed until it becomes a virtuous circle: in fact, the perception of the image of ourselves is also influenced by our attitude and our mood.

When we look in the mirror we talk to ourselves, we make judgments, and feel sensations and emotions.

We have already spoken about how to talk to ourselves in a better way, how to make our inner voice kinder and more respectful.

The essence of self-esteem is trusting your mind and knowing you can deserve happiness.
Nathaniel Branden (psychotherapist)

The psychotherapist Nathaniel Branden, an authority in the field of studies on self-esteem, in his bestseller "The Six Pillars Of Self Esteem", identifies six guiding principles that lead us to evaluate ourselves better.

Here they are summarised:

1. Live consciously

To live consciously means to observe your thoughts and how they build moods. Understand your beliefs about yourselves and the world, your values, your quality and your goals: what is really important to you.

2. Accept yourself

Accept how you really are, both positive and negative/less pleasant qualities, without lying to yourself.

3. The sense of responsibility

Understand that you are fully responsible for yourself, your thoughts, moods, emotions, your actions and choices, your goals and your life.

4. Self-affirmation

Give importance to yourself and the others, with no fear of expressing your opinions, your values and feelings.

5. Set yourself a goal

To know yourself also means to fully develop and realise your goals, giving yourself a purpose in life according to your aptitudes, inclinations, and talents. And move towards them with patience, perseverance, and method.

6. Personal Integrity

Personal integrity means to be consistent with your values and principles and keep commitments with yourself and the others in order to achieve the goals you set yourself.

I advise you to reflect on these guiding principles and to apply them and increase self-esteem.

Meanwhile, you can do the following exercises to improve the perception you have of yourself and your mood.

Start now...

EXERCISE NO. 7: Compliments...!

1. Stand in front of the mirror and look at your face and your pimples
2. Observe your thoughts (your inner voice and the feedback it gives you) and the emotions that arise
3. Transform any sentence into a positive one: give yourself compliments out loud and with your head held high, with

courage and determination. Repeat and insist!

EXERCISE NO. 8: Compliments, again…!

1.   Stand in front of the mirror and look at yourself
2.   Think about your successes and goals you have achieved so far (graduation, assignments, etc.)
3.   Think about how you got there, to your talents, your strengths…
4.   Think that no one is perfect but each of us has qualities… and you do too…

What we can do to further improve our mood and how we see ourselves?

First of all, "straight back"…
Our attitudes and moods are also manifested in our facial expression and in our body posture: if you feel sad, you will have a sad face, your back will be slightly bent, your head and your look facing down. This body attitude amplifies and reinforces the corresponding mood.

Certain facial expressions or postures can strengthen one state of mind but they can also change it.

If you feel sad or frustrated, it is because you are saying negative words to yourself and you have a certain posture or facial expression.
Try to change those words, your posture and your facial expression, and your mood will change: at first, just a little, then it
will progressively become easier and more effective as you practice.

EXERCISE 9: Are you sad and disappointed?

1.   stand in front of the mirror with your back straight
2.   put your head up
3.   look into your eyes
4.   smile to yourself: I know, you might find it difficult or stupid, but try to smile – the more you do it, the easier it will become.
5.   feel how the state of sadness decreases and changes

Lack of exercise and spending entire days watching TV and eating junk food is
typical of melancholy and depression.
You should not build or reinforce these habits.
You should turn the tide!

EXERCISE NO. 10: When you are feeling down..

When you feel down, if possible, stand in front of the mirror (it is necessary in order to appreciate and love yourself).
Do some of the following exercises:
1. twenty push-ups
2. twenty standing jumps
3. with your arms, simulate swimming
4. dance to the beat of your favourite songs
5. smile and sing out loud with no fear
6. do everything together

Try it!

How is your mood? Any better?
As I will explain later, exercising is a powerful antidote to sadness and depression: it helps to work off tension and release endorphins, the hormones of wellness and good mood.
And, as we have seen, all this is also good for pimples!

MANAGING STRESS

The skin is a thin sheet of tissue that covers the body. Physiologically, it is a rather simple organ; from psychological and social point of view, instead, it is a highly complex organ. The skin is a boundary between the outside and inside world, between the environment and yourself.
David Le Breton (Anthropologist)

As previously mentioned, stress is one of the secondary factors in the development of acne.

Through neuro-hormonal mechanisms, stress can lead to acne or to a worsening of it.

The psychosomatic dermatology is a super-specialist branch of dermatology who studies the relationship between mind and skin conditions. After all, in the human embryo, the nervous system and skin derive from the same cell lines; they have a common origin.

Also for this reason, there are complex interactions between psyche, nervous system, immune system, hormonal glands and skin: the psycho-neuro-immune-endocrine-cutaneous system is a just a little complicated way of saying that everything is connected, that our mind, our thoughts and feelings can affect the wellbeing (and beauty) and the state of disease (and inflammation) of our skin.

Sometimes, we are not even aware of our negative mood and our stress level, but they can worsen or cause acne, as well as trigger or worsen hives, psoriasis, and other dermatitis.

That is why it is important to learn how to manage stress.

What is stress, really?

The term stress was used for the first time by the physiologist Hans Selye (of Austrian origins) in 1936, in the journal called "Nature". He can be considered as the father of stress research.

According to Selye, stress is "the non-specific answer of the organism to each stimulus".

These stimuli could undermine the internal balance by inducing a situation of crisis, when you are unable to cope with them.

In his studies, he showed how animals exposed to prolonged stress were more likely to become ill.

The stress reaction manifests in three phases.

In the first phase, defined as **alarm** phase, the organism reacts with production of adrenaline (**fight or escape reaction**) – it is very similar to a state of anxiety (increased heart rate and blood sugar, faster breathing, the blood mainly flows to muscles).

Then comes the phase of **resistance or adaption**: the organism can cope or tends to adapt to the stressful situation and the physical reactions tend to normalise.

In the case in which the body is unable to adapt or overcome the stressful problem, it reaches the third phase, the **exhaustion** phase, where there is a psychophysical imbalance caused by the prolongation of the stressful situation.

As previously stated, chronic stress activates the adrenal glands and consequently increases the secretion of cortisol. If this hormone, also known as the stress hormone, is present in greater amounts, it can causes various problems: a general feeling of fatigue, increased heart rate (tachycardia), difficulty concentrating, frustration, irritability, anxiety, crying spells, sleep disturbances, confusion, boredom or hyperactivity, hyperglycemia and diabetes, widespread pain, colitis, gastritis and ulcers, lower immune response, and great susceptibility to illness.

However, stress is not always negative. Selye was also the first to distinguish two different types of stress, which he called distress or negative stress or eustress and positive stress.

Distress is just bad stress, the one which causes psychological and physical imbalances: it occurs when we fail to overcome the stressful situation due to several reasons:

1. **we do not have the ability or the appropriate skills** (e.g. an accident, surgery, disease, examination or race for which we are not prepared, a dismissal, a rejection, etc.)
2. **we overestimate the situation or the problem** although we can overcome it or underestimate **our abilities and skills**: we then feel helpless and do nothing to solve it.

Chronic diseases are often a source of distress regardless their severity.

Skin diseases are often chronic and although sometimes they are not severe or debilitating from a physical point of view, they affect the image of the individual and represent a chronic stressful situation for him/her.

This also applies to acne, where you can combine the two factors: it is objectively a chronic disease (but we can cure it) and it is often subjectively overestimated or the chances of winning against it are underestimated.

Prolonged exposure to a distress situation can cause the onset of both physical and psychological diseases (such as anxiety disorders), leading to a vicious circle that tends to prolong the state of stress.

The mental and physical balance is compromised and the effects of stress persist even in the absence of stressful events, or the body disproportionately reacts to other stimuli because of the anxious state – even if minor.

In fact, stress and anxiety are always closely related and anxiety tends to amplify the perception of potential hazard even in situations which are objectively normal.

The eustress or good stress, instead, can be defined it as the "spice of life".

When we are in our *"comfort zone"*, there is no stress because the environmental stimuli can be easily overcome as we have the ability and skills to do so.

When environmental stimuli push us to the limits or just outside of our "comfort or safety zone" and our capabilities are not yet sufficient to overcome them, eustress occurs. The stressful situation, but within our reach with a greater effort and commitment, leads us to further develop our abilities and improve ourselves in order to adapt to it.

The "adrenaline rush" increases comprehension and concentration, makes us decide rapidly, puts our muscles in a position to move quickly to attack, fight or fly, to have energy suitable to act in order to reach a goal more easily.

An example of eustress can be an intense work engagement, preparing for an assignment of a subject that we are passionate about, a job promotion: all this can bring benefits in terms of self-esteem, growth and self-realisation.

Additionally setting ourselves an "almost unachievable" goal can mean creating a positive stressor because it pushes us to get out of our comfort zone and to achieve it by developing our skills.

A certain amount of eustress allows us to have an active, rich and motivated life, with successes and failures.

Each of us constantly faces problems in life; it is a natural and normal "stressful" state.

Life is made up of events: from the single cell to the most complex cell system represented by an organism, every living being faces risks and obstacles at every moment.

The stimulus/event does not create stress!
Our limitations, skills or our assessments of the stimulus/event do!

Indeed, each of us responds to stressful events in a different way, because each person has different experiences, beliefs and abilities, and therefore interprets every single event differently.

It is also a question of learning i.e. the learnt attitude or choices: I act like this because I have learnt to react like this and I have always reacted like this.

These mechanisms become automatic, they go beyond our awareness.

However, between the stimulus and our reaction/response, we have always the possibility to choose how to assess the situation and how to react.

In any case, if we can see the event as a **potential insuperable hazard** then we will **experience a negative stress reaction** with all its consequences.

Or we can assess the situation as a challenge that we can win with our already acquired skills or to be acquired while we face it; we will use all our energies and do everything to face it as best as we can. And the stress will be positive. Think of all those times when obstacles and stressful situations seemed dangerous or insurmountable but in the end you successfully managed to face them thanks to your willpower, determination, and endurance.

Did you feel proud of yourself? How much?
Did your self-esteem improve? How much?

In order to effectively manage stress, you also need learn to manage anxiety, overcome fear, react positively to failure, and not fall after an error.

It is important to learn not to exaggerate problems and obstacles!

In acne in particular, I know that it is a problem that will create stress and anxiety and a subsequent vicious cycle (acne-stress-anxiety-stress-worsening of pimples) where you can remain trapped. Realising that effective treatments exist and committing to this 7 steps path already means to stop this mechanism. And it is already a step further: you can see your goal, a face free from pimples, as a challenge that you can face and overcome with no stress.

How to avoid negative stress or turn it into positive stress?

Evaluate the potential stressful problem, analyse it in all aspects by asking yourself these questions:

- what can it be helpful for?
- what skills can I gain if I face it and solve it?
- is it really insurmountable?
- have other people already faced it and solved it?
- have I already dealt with similar situations?
- are there different solutions to overcome it?

How do you relate to the problem?

- do you feel helpless?
- do you feel like a victim of the situation?
- do you think you do not have the ability or skills to solve it?
- are you pessimistic?

Martin Seligman, a professor of psychology at the University of Pennsylvania and bestselling author of "Learned optimism", is considered the founder of Positive Psychology and the pioneer of the studies of optimism and pessimism.

Depending on the behaviour, Seligman divides individuals into two categories: the optimists and the pessimists.

Pessimistic individuals manifest an attitude powerlessness and victimhood.

As we already know, attitudes are built by beliefs, assessments, and thoughts.

Each individual uses a particular way of thinking in order to interpret the daily events of his/her life: this is critical to direct his/her mood towards optimism or pessimism.

Life presents the same obstacles and tragedies to optimists and pessimists, but optimists face them better

Martin Seligman (psychologist)

Seligman has identified three key elements of the way that pessimists think when faced with unwanted potentially stressful events and formulated the theory of 3 P:

1. *Personalisation* (**it is my fault** if the situation is like this. I am not able)
2. *Permanence* (the situation will be **always like this**, long-lasting and persistent. I will never succeed.).
3. *Pervasiveness* (**everything** is going wrong and it will always go wrong).

These are generalisations which show that the glass is always half empty.

Therefore, **pessimists**:

- appear doubtful and hesitant when facing various events
- often assess problems as threats
- have little confidence in the possibility to overcome a problem or get the desired result
- often give up and do not face problems
- feel powerless to obstacles

Do you recognise yourself in this description, if you consider the way you deal with problems in general and your pimples?

In regards to these modes of thought, optimists generalise in the opposite direction and are more flexible, so they can see the glass half full.

Optimists

- tend to be confident and determined
- evaluate adversity as challenges to accept and win
- accept possible insurmountable limits in the external situation or the limitations of their abilities
- actively seek to solve problems and overcome difficulties

Overcoming adversity and achieving the desired goal, the optimists increase self-esteem and personal effectiveness.

Optimism is a state of mind determined by how a person explains and interprets the events that happen.
Martin Seligman (psychologist)

Martin Seligman also tells us that "the habits of thought should not last forever. People can choose their own way of thinking.
Indeed, pessimists can learn to be optimistic.

WHAT DO YOU NEED TO DO, IF YOU THINK NEGATIVELY?

1) Go against the 3 P (personalisation, permanence and pervasiveness), questioning the pessimistic generalisations and "eliminating" the negative way of thinking negatively:

<u>Eliminate personalisation:</u>
*It is **always all** your fault?*
*Are there **external factors** that prevent you to objectively solve the problem?*
*Have you **ever** successfully overcome a similar situation?*
*How could you **acquire or further develop the skills useful** for overcoming the challenge?*

<u>Remove the permanence:</u>
*How do you know that **everything will always go wrong**?*
*Has the situation **always been like that** or have there been phases of improvement when you were closer to solve the problem?*
*Have **already** successfully dealt with similar situations?*

<u>Remove the pervasiveness:</u>
*Is **everything** going wrong or is there something going well?*

*How do you know that **everything else** will go wrong?*
*In **what other situations** are you now solving problems?*
*In **what other situations** did you happily solve problems?*

2) When you realise that you are thinking negatively, observe and accept these thoughts without judgment and ask yourself:

What are these thoughts? What images, sounds, voices and feelings do these thoughts form?
How can I change these images, sounds, voices and feelings to see the problem from a different perspective?
What meaning or what other meanings can this problem have?
In a different context or situation, could the problem also have a different meaning or value?

Is there any situation or problem that I have not yet resolved and that causes this kind of thoughts?
How can I deal with and solve this problem? What skills or resources do I need to solve it?
And how can I acquire them?

These questions will lead you to reflect on your attitudes towards situations and problems that you encounter. Acne is an objectively stressful problem: however, a more positive and optimistic attitude will help reduce stress and to solve it better, with more confidence and determination.

OPTIMISM and STRESS

Cortisol is the hormone produced in response to anxiety and chronic stress, and we already know the harmful effects that its persistent increase causes on health in general and acne in particular.

Normally, it quickly increases in the morning, at 8 am, and then begins to decrease until it stabilises at minimum levels at around midnight.

If a person is stressed out, cortisol in the morning will be above the physiological level, with a consequent increase in blood sugar (during fasting). This causes an increase in insulin which stimulates further secretion of cortisol.

Relaxation and meditation and self-awareness techniques reduce the level of cortisol and increase the secretion of endorphins: hormones which create the feeling of wellbeing.

Moreover, many studies have observed that, in the morning, the optimists produce less cortisol, are healthier, live a more fulfilling life, and are happier.

more optimism = less stress = less cortisol = less inflammation = more wellbeing and happiness

As you will see later, a happier life leads us to reach our goals more easily, improve our health and our wellbeing, whilst minimising all physical and psychic toxins that contribute to the worsening of pimples.

STEP III: THE DERMATOLOGIST

If you regularly do the exercises that I proposed in the first two steps in order to support and strengthen your determination to achieve the ultimate goal, you can start with step III.

Now the basic **skills** to develop or improve are:

- how to choose your dermatologist
- how to prepare yourself to the dermatological examination

in order to achieve the **intermediate goals**:

- perform an effective dermatological examination
- set treatments with your dermatologist

You will choose the dermatologist to begin dermatological and outpatient treatments, go towards a marked improvement and finally have your pimples under control.

THE DERMATOLOGIST AND THE DERMATOLOGICAL EXAMINATION

There is a lot of misinformation circulating; many people (either professionals or not) often propose miraculous treatments for acne. And, understandably, you may be wondering:

should I go to the dermatologist to treat acne?

The dermatologist is the skin specialist: he/she has extensively studied its structure, how it works, and different diseases including acne. With experience, he/she has developed the so-called "clinical eye" and knowledge of therapies and their effects, as well as cosmetics and their potential benefits.

Sometimes you find the right dermatologist, try to follow a treatment, but after two weeks (or maybe two months) you do not see any results and you might think that you should contact another specialist:

- *the dermatologist was not the right one?*
- *the treatment was not effective?*
- *you were expecting more rapid improvements or definitive result?*

If you are serious about defeating pimples, you need the support of a good dermatology specialist who will recommend you the most appropriate treatment for the type of acne you are suffering from.

Of course, he should also be an expert in the treatment of acne and have excellent knowledge in cosmetology.

There are also other factors to carefully consider for the final choice of your dermatologist.

HOW TO CHOOSE YOUR DERMATOLOGIST

Before booking an appointment it is good to ask some questions:

1. *Is he/she a real expert in anti-acne treatments?*
2. *How long is his/her experience in the field?*
3. *What is your friends' or relatives' opinion? Have they benefited from the recommended treatment?*

The dermatologist does not need to be "famous"; he/she should have good reputation among acquaintances, on the web, in your city.

Once you have chosen and contacted the dermatologist, the day of the dermatological examination finally arrives.

Yes, you are also responsible for the outcome of the consultation: you will need to be prepared for it as you will have to actively participate.

HOW TO PREPARE FOR THE DERMATOLOGICAL EXAMINATION

As yourself the following questions that the dermatologist will surely ask you:

- what treatments have you followed so far? What are the results?
- are your menstrual cycles regular?
- what are your cosmetic habits?
- what cosmetic products have you used in the last few months?
- what cosmetic products are you currently using?
- have you done any outpatient treatment (peeling, photodynamic, etc.)? What are the results?

Have a good think and:

A. make a list of cosmetic products you are using for your face: from lotions to moisturisers and make-up products. You can bring packaging where it is possible to read the ingredients.
B. make a list of the dermatological treatments followed in the past and more recently.
C. remember if you made outpatient treatment: when, how, what kind?
D. if you had blood tests or hormonal assays done, bring the results with you.

Remember: the more you are clear in providing data, the more the dermatologist will treat your acne better.

Together you can analyze the story of your acne and evaluate the importance of the various causative factors in the formation of your pimples; every case is different and everyone needs a personalised approach and therapy.

Furthermore:
- *what type of skin do you think you have?*
- *do you think you have sensitive or delicate skin?*

Finally, what do you expect from the dermatologist's prescription?

a) a definitive healing from acne?
b) a significant improvement in just one week?
c) a gradual improvement in a few weeks?
d) complicated and expensive treatment?
e) general treatment with many side effects?

It is necessary to have your ideas clear about your expectations and objectives so that you can discuss and share them with the dermatologist during the examination.

In this way, you will not have doubts; you can get advice and guidance with confidence and start the treatment path with him/her.

ASSESSING THE DERMATOLOGIST

Although you expect the best from a professional, the dermatologist is not infallible and you should understand that he/she may have character limitations, be subject to errors and moments of tiredness like everyone else. Having said this, during the examination you should assess the way he/she approaches you and your condition:

A. ***Is he/she asking me if I have already followed other treatments and their results?***

B. *Is he/she underestimating the importance that **I give** to my pimples?*

C. ***Is he/she promising miraculous results proposing a "package" of fairly expensive treatments?***

D. *Or is he/she asking me to be patient and consistent because the therapy will be long-lasting and continuous? Is he/she asking me to take responsibility and follow the treatment at home? Is he/she advising the best treatment possible for me?*

E. ***Is he/she asking me about all cosmetics that I have used and I am using?***

F. Does he/she have a comprehensive approach? Is he/she sensitive to my impatience and my frustration? Is he/she really listening or does he/she constantly talk non-stop?

G. Is he/she explaining why he/she prescribes me certain products and bans or avoid other ones? Does he/she speak about possible problems and side effects that can occur with certain products or drugs?

H. Does he/she make sure if I have understood the therapy? Does he/she try to clear all my doubts?

I. Does he/she look for my cooperation and "partnership" in fighting pimples or does he/she just hands me a list of products to use?

J. Does he/she explains how "we will get there"?

If the answer to most of these questions is yes, you should be in good hands and you have probably found a dermatologist who will follow you to the fullest.

It is really important to rely on an experienced dermatologist who can guide you in treating acne and that is able to personalise the therapy.

But it is even more important that you understand that a good percentage of the success of anti-acne treatments and the fight against pimples depends on you!

The dermatologist can prescribe and set the best anti-acne treatment, but that means nothing if you do not implement it or if you follow it only partially or irregularly!

It is totally up to you to choose to follow it... with patience and perseverance.

- set intermediate goals with your dermatologist
- be ready to implement the necessary changes to the therapy
- be precise in following the instructions: rushing can lead to irritation and needs a temporary suspension of care
- do not be discouraged if you see an initial decline, it may happen sometimes. Inform the specialist.

The fight against pimples is a marathon: it takes time.

THE 5 CONDITIONS TO WIN AGAINST ACNE

1. It is important to tell your dermatologist about all therapies, cosmetics and treatments for pimples followed in the past.

Once again, during the dermatological examination, it will be useful to highlight everything that has given some degree of improvement, a moment worsening or what it turned to be useless.

You should also tell the dermatologist about all remedies for pimples that you have used, including medications that you are taking for other health problems.

A good dermatologist wants to have this information and will ask you a lot of questions.

2. The dermatologist will be your best ally.

You might have had bad experiences in the past: treatments did not work, doctors or dermatologists who did not follow you as you wanted or how you thought he/she should have.

Do not expect that the dermatological examination, the prescription or the anti-acne treatment are able to eliminate pimples. Only you can do that, if the treatment is right, and with the help of the dermatologist.

3. Improving acne takes time.

I know, you are looking forward to eliminating pimples and finally having smooth, clean and normal skin again. Unfortunately, no treatment or drug acts in one day: you must be patient.

In the best case scenario, if the prescribed anti-acne treatment is adequate and you skin responds well to it, in 10-15 days, you should already notice an improvement: the inflammation is reduced and pimples become less red and less painful.

In most cases, it takes about 1 month to see the first benefits of the treatment.

4. Perseverance is key!

The dermatologist's task is to advise the best cure for pimples and your skin, explain how to use the products, when applying them during the day, and inform you on what cosmetics to avoid.

But your job is to precisely follow the treatment: apply the anti-acne products and take the prescribed medications regularly.

Poor results of a treatment are often just due to the irregular or wrong application of the products: if something is not clear or if you have problems, please contact your dermatologist. A good dermatologist wants you contact him/her in case of doubts.

5. **The final goal: normalising the skin and have acne under control.**

The first month of acne therapy is crucial. It is often necessary to adjust the treatment pattern to fit the response of your skin: no cosmetic product or medication is good for all skin types, the effects can vary.

After the improvement, it is necessary to aim at normalising acne: acne cannot be cured, but it can be effectively kept under control, having the skin clean, free from blackheads and pimples.

This result can be achieved only by following the treatments, even when pimples have almost completely disappeared: the dermatologist will guide you reducing products to use and making the anti-acne therapy easier.

TEST NO. 3 - ACNE FORECASTS

When we start the anti-acne treatment, we often would like to know where we are and what comes next: how many pimples will appear or disappear in the coming weeks or months.

The dermatologist can often give us a prediction on the appropriate time needed before seeing the first benefits of the treatment that he/she prescribed to you.

An effective therapy for acne rarely begins to show improvements after a few days; it more often happens after several weeks: pimples, papules and inflamed pustules begin to dry out and become less inflamed until they disappear – and they will probably leave red or dark acne spots.

In any case, new pimples continue to appear and acne seems invincible.

It is normal for pimples to continue to form, do not get discouraged.

The important thing is to look at the trend, the overall trend: day by day, week by week, **does the number of pimples that constantly appear tend to diminish?**

What else can be a sign of worsening (or improvement)?
How can you predict how many pimples will appear in the coming weeks?

Examine your skin and evaluate **the number and density of comedones.**

Most of them will become pimples in a time ranging from a few days to a few weeks.

Compared to when you started the anti-acne therapy:

- *has the overall number of comedones decreased or increased?*
- *has the density of comedones, in the various areas of the face, decreased or increased?*

This is the fundamental data!

It is important to observe in particular **the depth of whiteheads** (pimples under the skin) because, according to their depth, you will be able to roughly predict how long you will need to wait before you have a cleaner skin.

Whiteheads will inevitably originate as waves of deep pimples, which can leave some real holes in the skin.

Stretch your skin with your fingers:
- *if you have any, do deep whiteheads become more visible?*
- *are there still many of them?*

N.B. This test is for guidance only. Diagnosis and treatment of acne and its outcomes are the sole responsibility of your doctor and must necessarily be tailored and adapted to the clinical picture.

STEP IV: SKIN CARE AND TREATMENT

Everything should be made as simple as possible, but not simpler.
Albert Einstein (physicist)

THE LESS THE BETTER

I often see people with acne who have followed many treatments and are discouraged by the lack or scarcity of results. They often have consulted more doctors, dermatologists, and aestheticians but have not seen great benefits.

I also see people fighting pimples following advice from friends and relatives, popular magazines, with "do it yourself" treatments that not only failed to eliminate pimples but also led to a worsening of acne.

It is true that when somebody is desperately searching for the right acne treatment, they make many attempts, they make a "botch" of it or come across "natural cures" that they regret later on...

In order to cure acne, I always thought that what we apply on our skin is as equally important as what we do not apply.

I have always believed that, in most cases, our skin has its own ability to defend itself, rebalance and rejuvenate. Then the studies, practice and experience have confirmed this.

My patients with acne are often surprised, sometimes incredulous, about my prescription.

With 2-3 products, will the anti-acne treatment be really effective?
I have used so many with no results and now I should use so few of them?

I tell them to trust me and be patient because the rush to win against acne only leads them to make mistakes.

Then, when I explain why using less products is better, that sometimes even just using a cleanser suitable for their skin can already show a certain degree of improvement, and that it is better not to make a mess of it and make the acne more inflamed, they understand and follow with the method the therapy for acne that I recommended.

And, as you will read, it is a therapy that is not limited to dermatological care, but it concerns small and gradual changes of cosmetic and dietary habits and lifestyle.

They come back to me even more surprised, but happy for the benefits gained. They seem to be reborn, more optimistic and feel how they should feel at their age: they have recovered or are recovering the loss of self-esteem and self-confidence.

They are indeed even more determined to keep their skin clean and free from pimples!

When the anti-acne treatment works, a virtuous circle is established: a gradual reduction of pimples and a healthier skin push the patient to follow the advice and the prescriptions with more confidence and perseverance. And this, in turn, leads to a further improvement.

As previously mentioned about the acne-stress-anxiety-depression correlation, seeing yourself improving also determines hormonal changes, with additional benefits.

As you might have noticed, I dedicated an entire chapter about this aspect, which is very important but underestimated by traditional dermatology.

The chapter has to do with the true and ultimate purpose for which patients with acne desperately want to defeat it: living the most beautiful season of their lives better and with joy!

QUICK REMEDIES FOR PIMPLES? No thanks!

Discovering rapid treatments for pimples in order to say goodbye to acne is the dream of dermatologists and patients.

There are many websites and online articles about rapid treatment for pimples, scars and spots from acne, but if you read carefully, they often promote products or instrumental treatments, more or less expensive, that promise miraculous results.

Unfortunately there are no miracles, nor on the web nor in reality.

I do not want you to feel discouraged now (maybe you already do), but, unfortunately, in order to win your war against pimples, you first need to face the truth: acne treatments are long and you need to have patience and perseverance.

This does not mean that you cannot see improvements in a short time.

The message I want to convey is that your approach to the anti-acne treatment is as critical as the treatment itself, if you want to obtain good results and keep acne under control.

It all starts with the right attitude and the right motivation!

When you are fighting pimples, it is important to be wary of remedies for pimples that promise rapid and perhaps definitive healing.

Instead, you should:
- be methodical
- think about the medium-term results
- never get discouraged and give up
- never rush or be desperate and try all remedies for pimples and various advertised cosmetics as per word-of-mouth from friends or relatives: the risk is a worsening of your acne!

THE BEST TIME TO TREAT PIMPLES

Here it comes: the day when you have had enough and decide that it is time to treat your condition for real.

As previously mentioned, fighting pimples requires commitment, but also a strategy and a specific timetable, if you want to see results.

You cannot go by trial and error: try a product, then another, then a treatment and so on. By doing so, you lose time and money, and in the meantime your acne might worsen.

Treating acne is a path to start and continue with perseverance and patience.

Autumn and winter is the best time to start treating acne.

In fact, you can use drugs or cosmetics that you can hardly apply during summer and you will be able to undergo treatments that are not doable in the late spring or summer.

Only in autumn and winter you can use the best acne treatments:

- **retinoids** (such as tretinoin and adapalene) with restructuring and exfoliating action progressively reduce existing comedones (whiteheads and blackheads) and slow down the formation of new ones keeping pores free and clean.
- **benzoyl peroxide**, with antiseptic and exfoliating action, quickly dries pimples and reduces blackheads.
- **antibiotics** (such as tetracyclines) with antibacterial and anti-inflammatory action reduce existing pimples and acne inflammation.

And the most effective treatment for acne: the **chemical peel**: a technique which uses the application of acid to the skin in order to quickly dry out pimples and eliminate blackheads and whiteheads, leading to an exfoliation and to a real deep cleansing of the skin.

It is an extremely powerful outpatient treatment, adjustable to the type of acne you are suffering from: 1-2 peeling sessions can provide benefits comparable to about two months of home therapies.

All of these products and treatments are very effective, and you have to take into account slight irritation or dryness of the skin, if you want to follow anti-acne treatments that give results. However, they can also be very abrasive or favour the appearance of pimples when the heat and the sun are intense.

You decide if it is better for you to wait or reach the summer with a face already cleaner and free from pimples.

Please note, if you happen to read this book during summer: I am not saying to postpone everything after the summer season. Contact your dermatologist and start treatments immediately.

The sooner you start treating pimples, the better.
The fact that therapies cannot be aggressive does not mean that they will not benefit you.

Even with less aggressive therapies, you will begin your path to the final goal: to put acne under control and have a clear skin.

In any case, with appropriate treatments, your skill will rebalance and become less inflamed, and even the sun and the sea will be of help. Start, and then launch the decisive attack on the pimples in the autumn-winter.

THE 4 PILLARS OF AN EFFECTIVE ANTI-ACNE TREATMENT
The virtuous circle of anti-acne therapy

Making the simple complicated is commonplace; making the complicated simple, awesomely simple, that's creativity.
Charles Mingus (musician)

In the first part of this book, I briefly described how and why acne manifests. Perhaps you felt a little discouraged to see what and how many causes contribute to the formation of pimples, the complexity of mechanisms, and what and how many forms of acne there are.

In fact, looking at them one by one, these factors are numerous and appear to be complex because they are intertwined and affect each other.

But if we look at the whole, we can also see that there are common factors; there is a same global underlying mechanism where local factors might come into play and trigger the inflammatory process of acne.

It is important to know the mechanisms that produce pimples and understand upon which ones we can act in order to finally tackle acne and put it under control.

As you will see, having identified and fully understood these mechanisms, you will become aware that you can do it and that we can make the anti-acne treatments simpler, faster and, above all, effective. Now, let us move on and learn what we should act upon in order to stop, reverse and turn these pathological

mechanisms into virtuous circles so that we determine a progressive and steady improvement.

Because it is not only about drying out pimples and making them less inflamed, but acting further upstream: the therapy should not be a temporary expedient, just to provide some relief, but it should aim to restore skin balance so that the formation of blackheads and pimples is reduced.

My method to treat acne is based on 4 strategic activities on which the patient should focus simultaneously and synergistically, if he/she wants to achieve a global impact on acne disease:

1.   Cleanse to rebalance
2.   Turn off the inflammation
3.   Exfoliate to clean deeply
4.   Keep the results

Just as the factors which cause acne are linked together in a tight and complex way, these points cannot be considered individually; they are closely related as well and strengthen each other, thus creating a balancing virtuous circle.

In fact, it is important to highlight that if we focus on just one or two of these points, treatments will give temporary or poor benefits: even if you neglect one of them, the impact of anti-acne therapy will be reduced and you will not be able to globally tackle acne.

Therefore, think about these activities as the construction of a circular and self-reinforcing path, **_the virtuous anti-acne circle_**, in which we start from adequate cleansing, then we add the

neutralisation of inflammatory processes and finally the exfoliation. This is the only way we can achieve the final goal: the normalisation of the skin, which is a result that we will need to maintain in order to feed the virtuous circle of the skin free from pimples that responds better to therapies. And therapies will then become more and more effective, simple, and minimal.

The virtuous anti-acne circle

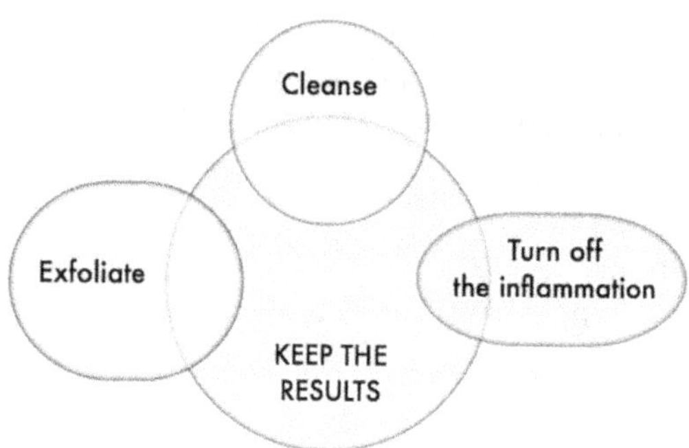

CLEANSE TO REBALANCE

Cleansing has a vital role in keeping the skin healthy and, therefore, in treating acne as well: we can follow the best anti-acne treatment in the world, but if we do not clean the skin properly, we will not get the desired benefits.

Cleansers may contain chemicals such as surfactants or oils able to catch dirt and sebum, allowing you to remove them with water.

The more the foam is produced, the greater the washing and degreasing power... And the irritating power!

And we know that acneic skin is already irritated enough, so you should not use a product that further aggravates this irritation. You should instead choose a product that is going to reduce it.

The secret lies in respecting the skin balance.

We often read or they tell us that the act of cleansing the skin and remove impurities, excess sebum, smog and dirt is important, but what makes the difference is how we do it!

If the goal is to degrease the skin to get rid of unpleasant and annoying shiny appearance, then an effective cleanser can be ethyl alcohol (or perhaps acetone...): the skin will certainly look clean, fresh, and smooth immediately... But later on? In fact, after just 1 hour, it will become much glossier and greasier than it was before. You could then insist, as they told you that oily skin needs to be cleaned, but after a few days, you would see a significant worsening of the glossy aspect of your skin.

This is the so-called rebound effect: **the more you degrease your skin, the more it becomes fatty and greasy!** The more you insist on washing your face and the quicker it becomes shiny.

The problem is the cleanser that you arc using!

Maybe you are using a special cleanser for acne because you have some pimples and you were told that degreasing your skin also dries out pimples.

It is true, you will immediately feel like your skin is cleaner, with improved papules and pustules, but if the cleanser (although being labelled as "for acne") is not really the right one for your type of acne and skin, after just a few hours or days the pimples might be even more inflamed ... And your skin might be even oilier.

The ideal cleanser should therefore:

1.   only partially remove the sebum on the surface: the amount in excess
2.   not alter the acidic pH (5 to 5.5) of the skin
3.   not eliminate or alter the hydrolipidic film by removing the sebum and other components

Furthermore, an ideal cleanser for acne should contain:

4.   soothing and sebum-normalising substances that reduce acne inflammation and, gradually, the sebaceous secretion.

TURN OFF THE INFLAMMATION

In the past, it was believed that acne inflammation was mainly due to the bacterial factor, which considered Propionibacterium acnes (PA) as the main one. This belief is apparently still confirmed by the effectiveness of (local and general) antibiotic treatments aimed at reducing inflammation and improving acne.

As the knowledge of the molecular biochemistry of inflammation has expanded with the discovery of the role of free radicals and eicosanoids, Propionibacterium acnes has been partially cleared.

The fact that PA proliferates within the occluded follicle is a consequence of the occlusion itself, as I explained earlier.

The PA itself does not cause acne and its contribution to inflammation is almost zero during the initial phase (comedogenesis). It later becomes greater, but always in relative terms.

We have seen that the acne inflammation is caused by factors such as:

- Free radicals: lipoperoxides
- Immune reaction to Propionibacterium acnes
- Immune reaction to sebum leaking into the dermis

These act locally and quickly.

It is also favoured and supported by secondary general factors:

- Imbalanced diet, with high glycemic index foods and omega 3 deficiency
- Chronic stress

which contribute to the overall level of silent chronic inflammation, i.e. "the level of the tide". These factors act more subtly and require changes in your lifestyle. They will benefit you more deeply and less visibly, but only in the medium-long term.

EXFOLIATE TO CLEAN DEEPLY

As previously stated, cleansing is a fundamental act for restoring the balance of your skin but it is certainly not enough. It is not enough to halt acne inflammation.

The inflamed pimples are just the tip of the iceberg of the acne process. In the chapter about the 4 primary causes of acne, I explained that ache all starts with the occlusion of the pilosebaceous follicle and the formation of the comedo.

Comedones form at the epidermis level and therefore you need aim at the epidermis normalisation: the ideal goal of an effective treatment is to bring comedones formation to zero.

They are the fundamental lesions that are always present in any type of acne; they originate all future pimples.

The problem lies in the comedones!

Look at the skin of your face, the comedones that you see will soon be pimples, if you do not begin to treat them.

It is easy and normal to squeeze a blackhead: in this way, the trapped sebum comes out and the pore remains dilated, you have temporarily solved the problem but that does not prevent the pore from becoming blocked and the blackhead from forming again.

In people suffering from acne or with oily skin, blackheads and whiteheads tend to form regularly. You cannot permanently eliminate them, but you can prevent them: you can eliminate the causes that lead to their formation so that the number of them is progressively reduced until they disappear completely.

Only this will lead to a smaller number of pimples and to an overall improvement of your acne.

Eliminating them means to normalise the skin and put the acne disease under control.

Therefore, we need to act on the ductal hyperkeratosis.

A goal that you can set in the first 4 weeks is to reduce the formation of horny plugs at the pores level and liberate the majority of those already clogged.

We can achieve this goal by accelerating the turnover of epidermal cells and "dissolving" the horny plugs.

The epidermis regenerates every 28 days.

We can act on clogged pores with products containing exfoliating active ingredients (hydroxy acids, retinoids, etc.): they can act through different mechanisms, but their final effect is the exfoliation.

But what is exfoliation? How does it work?

This term indicates the detachment of the cells of the stratum corneum (the outermost layer of the epidermis) or even of the deepest epidermal layers (spinous layer and basal layer). If it only concerns the stratum corneum, it is called superficial exfoliation (almost invisible). It is clear that there are different levels of exfoliation.

As previously mentioned, it is the final effect of the various exfoliating substances. As you will see, these can have other effects that treat acne with varying levels of success.

Here is the general rule:
the deeper (within given limits) the exfoliation, the greater the benefits.

With exfoliation, we obtain the removal of the "horny plug" which occludes the pore. And with continuous exfoliation, we prevent the stratum corneum from excessive thickening (hyperkeratosis) at the level of the follicular duct: the horny cells do not remain attached to the surface, but they flake and "fall like leaves".

The secret of an effective anti-acne therapy is to achieve this goal: to eliminate comedones.

This is only possible with exfoliation!

Of course, the effects will not be immediate, you will need to wait for a few weeks before seeing your skin cleaner.

If you desire more immediate results, and if there is an active acne, you can also have a few sessions of peeling or exfoliating fractional radiofrequency: your skin will look cleaner after the first session and even the exfoliating cosmetics used at home will be more effective.

As we will see in greater detail later, we can distinguish two types of exfoliation depending on the means that we use: chemical and mechanical.

For various reasons that we will cover later on, it is preferable to choose chemical exfoliation, as it is proven to be more effective.

KEEP THE RESULTS

You have seen an improvement and then, after some time, even pimples are gone: the skin is smooth and clean at last.

The treatment is the right one this time, it is now time to finally stop applying lotions and other products...

So you stop all treatment, for a few days you do not wash your face or you wash it with normal soap... Acne is finally defeated...

But within a few days, you start feeling your skin become less smooth, seeing some blackheads and then pimples reappear again.

You have let your guard down, but unfortunately you see that it is not over.

As previously explained, your skin is prone to acne or, more precisely, is designed to form blackheads and whiteheads. This predisposition will last forever, even though the influence of male hormones will progressively reduce after the peak of adolescence. In any case, acne indeed tends to improve with the passing of time.

If you think that you can beat acne in just a few weeks, you will be inevitably disappointed.

If an improvement occurs, the credit does not only go to the right treatment but also to you: you meticulously followed the therapy and you were determined and dedicated.

You must continue to treat your skin regularly.

When I talk about treatment, I do not necessarily mean a therapy with many drugs and anti-acne lotions. It may surprise you, but a cleanser should be enough sometimes, as long as it is appropriate. I think that treatments for pimples should be as simple and easy to follow as possible.

When, during a first examination with a patient, I read previous prescriptions with long lists of cleansers (medicated cleanser, cosmetic cleanser, make-up remover and toner), a cream for the night, one for the morning and another one for the afternoon, mask or scrub, make-up products, moisturisers, antibiotics and more, I understood why the patient did not follow the treatment and had no results.

It was a treatment that could hardly be beneficial because, despite all the good intentions, the action of some products inevitably cancels the action of others, as I will explain later.

It was a treatment that the patient was not able to follow and this is not his/her responsibility.

The improvement of your acne and skin normalisation is a goal that you can achieve in the short/medium term. Keeping the results is a long-term goal and it can only be achieved by further simplifying the therapy and making it become a normal daily routine.

The two secrets for winning against acne forever are: simplicity and perseverance.

HOME TREATMENTS

Home therapies include the set of medications and dermocosmetic products that the dermatologist prescribed to the patient to use at home.

They can be of two types:

- topical or external
- systemic or internal.

Topical therapies are those which are directly applied to the skin and include:

- dermocosmetic products
- drugs

while systemic therapies include:

a. general or systemic drugs
b. food supplements
c. diet

In case of acne, drugs are usually taken via oral route and, much more rarely, intramuscularly or intravenously.

As we will see later on, food supplements and diet play an important role in the medium/long term.

The next chapters will be dedicated to the three major typical groups of anti-acne dermatological treatments and relevant subgroups:

- dermocosmetic products
- topical drugs
- systemic drugs

In two other chapters we will describe the herbal remedies and the food supplements that could be complementary and useful in the anti-acne therapy.

I will describe their main characteristics, type and formulas. Bear in mind that knowing the anti-acne products, cosmetics or drugs, will prevent you from starting "do it yourself" therapies that might result ineffective or harmful. In order to set an anti-acne treatment (or any dermatological and medical treatment), you should always consult a dermatologist or your family doctor.

A very important rule is that **there cannot be a cure without a specific diagnosis**, i.e. an evaluation that necessarily happens in person during a medical or dermatological examination. And vice versa, any therapy that you follow, each product you use by hearsay or by the advice of friends or online consultants, cannot be accurate and correct. It is just a shortcut that can do damage or lead you astray, making you lose precious time.

We can classify acne products based on their action, which depends on their active ingredients.
And this classification is more useful to understand which causal factors of acne they act upon and what their role is in the therapeutic strategy.
As you will notice, these distinctions somehow stress the 4 strategic activities of the anti-acne virtuous circle that I mentioned earlier.
Here are the 5 major categories:

- Exfoliants
- Anti-inflammatory or soothing products
- Antiseptics
- Antibiotics
- Retinoids

DERMOCOSMETIC PRODUCTS

Once again, the dermocosmetic products and cosmetics you use are important: the success of the anti-acne treatment also depends on them.

Treating the skin with appropriate cosmetics can mark the boundary between a beautiful and healthy skin and an irritated and inflamed one, i.e. a ill skin.

The keyword is: balance.

The products that help maintain or restore balance promote the wellbeing of our skin.

What exactly is a cosmetic?

Here is what the Italian Law 713/86 say:
Art. 1
*1. For the purposes of this Regulation, 'cosmetic product' means any substance or mixture intended to be placed in contact with the various external parts of the human body (epidermis, hair system, nails, lips and external genital organs) or with the teeth and the mucous membranes of the oral cavity with a view exclusively or mainly to cleaning them, perfuming them, changing their appearance, protecting them, **keeping them in good condition** or correcting body odours.*
2. The cosmetic product has no therapeutic purpose or activity.

Reformulated in the subject of this book:

*for the Italian and European Regulation, a cosmetic product is any product which, when applied to the surface of the skin, helps to clean, moisturise, colour or decorate it, **protecting its balance and keeping it (at least) in good condition (and maybe) improving its health and wellbeing.***

Cosmetics are not drugs. Drugs are products that have a therapeutic activity and purpose, i.e. they cure the ill skins, in this case, skins with acne.

So, why do dermatologists often recommend cosmetics together with drugs?

They do because **cosmetics are rebalancing remedies for your**

skin.

As they are not drugs and free to be purchased, used and sometimes recommended without any scientific criteria, cosmetic products are often "underrated" in their function, leading to errors and abuse.

To advise and prescribe cosmetics, instead, requires careful assessment of skin type, skin disease or condition that you want to cure or adjust. In fact, there are many cosmetic products on the market and the likelihood that most of them are not suitable for our skin is very high. That is why I do not advise to use them via word of mouth, experience of friends or advertising.

This applies to any cosmetic product: it is very hard to find (and guess) the cosmetics suitable for our skin! It is often even complicated for the dermatologist because it is almost impossible to forecast how the skin of a person will react (positively and negatively) to the application and use of a given cosmetic product.

Dermatology and medicine are not exact sciences. There are no formulas or algorithms able to lead to certain results.

However, the competence of the dermatologist in cosmetology and the experience of many mistakes and successes give him/her the ability to predict what impact a given cosmetic product might have on a given type of skin.

If you are fighting your personal war against pimples, this is my message: going by trial and error and trying product by product seldom leads to benefits. It actually often leads to a significant and disastrous worsening of your acne.

In general, the cosmetic products used in acne can be divided into various types depending on their formula and function:

- **Cleansers**
- **Moisturisers**
- **Exfoliants**
- **Masks**
- **Mattifiers**
- **Cover creams**

Cleansers

Cleansing is the first step of any cosmetic routine.

The cleansers generally have the function to cleanse the skin by removing:

- excess sebum
- sweat
- dirt
- smog
- dead cells
- residues of make-up and other cosmetics
- possible harmful bacteria

They can act chemically and/or mechanically.

If we read the above list again, we can see that some substances are fat (e.g. sebum and the make-up residues) and others are aqueous (e.g. sweat).

We should consider cleansing as a predominantly chemical process: aqueous substances remove aqueous substances more easily and fatty substances combine with fatty substances, facilitating their removal from the skin surface.

Therefore, washing your face with water only would definitely remove sweat, but not sebum and make-up – and this would not be a complete cleaning.

We can smear and rub fatty and oily substances on the face to incorporate sebum and residues of make-up, but then... how do we remove everything? Sure, we could use cotton, but a part of it would inevitably remain on the surface of our skin, leaving it moisturised and also slightly greasy and shiny.

In both cases, we would not have the feeling of having a fresh and clean skin, would we?

Indeed, the real problem of cleansing is to remove grease effectively!

The fatty substances can be eliminated in three ways:

1. dissolving them with a solvent (alcohol)
2. mixing them with water (with the help of surfactants)
3. removing them via affinity (tying them to other fat)

As previously stated, if we use fatty and oily substances, we might not know how to remove everything from the skin.

If we use products containing alcohol solvents (e.g. alcohol toners or wipes made with isopropyl or ethyl alcohol), we would clean the skin too much, not only removing excess sebum but also much of the hydrolipidic film.

In fact, **cleansing must be effective, but also gentle**: it should respect the balance of your skin!

Here the surfactants come to play. They are "magic" chemical substances able to bind fatty substances and water together, forming a little or a lot of foam, allowing us to remove everything (fat and sweat) with a refreshing final rinse.

But... There are various types of surfactants, those that are more or less aggressive:

- Anionic
- Amphoteric
- Non-ionic

The last two groups are the most gentle and tolerated ones.

You might wonder, chemistry aside, how do I figure out if and how aggressive a cleanser is?

Look at the foam that the cleanser produces: the more the foam is produced, the greater the degreasing power – and higher is the unbalancing and irritating power.

A practical example, try to wash your hands with dish soap: can you see how much foam it produces? Rinse and dry your hands, do not you feel your skin clean but a little dry?

You would think that is precisely what you want: a perfectly clean and dry skin, with no grease and shiny appearance.

But then what?

We know that the acneic skin is already irritated enough so you should use a product that does not worsen the state of irritation. The product actually needs to reduce it!

There are various types of cleansers that can be grouped into the following categories:

- Soaps
- Non-soaps

- Rinse-off cleansing creams
- Cleansing milks (No rinse)
- Toners and astringents
- Micellar waters
- Exfoliants
- Scrubs or granular cleansers
- Cleansing or make-up removal wipes
- Cleansing masks

They can contain substances with exfoliating, soothing and antiseptic, and sebum normalising action.

Let us review the various types of cleanser; I will tell you which ones are better to use.

Soaps

Sodium soaps prepared from sodium hydroxide (caustic soda) are generally in solid form, while potassium soaps prepared from potassium hydroxide (caustic potash) are softer or often in liquid form.

In this category, the traditional soap is the most common, whether it is normal soap, Marseille soap or sulphur soap.

Traditional soap is made of sodium salts of fatty acids and consists of beef tallow (80%), refined animal fats and coconut oil or olive oil (20%).

The soaps produced from olive oil are softer and gentler, e.g. Marseille soap, well-known for its delicacy.

However, **soaps have a pH of 9 - 10.5 (alkaline)** and therefore they raise a lot the pH of the skin, which normally is 5 - 5.5.

This leads to a disruption of skin balance, with loss of the protective functions of the hydrolipidic film: reduction of bacteriostatic effect and increased irritability of the skin.

Moreover, in the presence of calcareous water, limestone salts form on the surface of the skin and lead to dryness and irritation.

Tip: to be avoided!

Non-soaps

There are also the so-called **acid soaps**, also called **non-soaps** or **synthetic detergent**.

They are divided into anionic, non-ionic and amphoteric.

They consist of mixtures of surfactants such as sodium lauryl sulphate or alkyl sulphonate surfactants, organic esters of sulphuric acid.

Such non-soaps have a pH of 5.5, similar to that of the skin, thus resulting less aggressive due to the absence of free alkalinity.

They are in liquid or gel form.

Tip: use non-soaps with amphoteric and nonionic surfactants. They are close to the ideal cleanser for oily and non-sensitive acne-prone skin.

Rinse-off cleansing creams

They are represented by rinse-off cream or cleansing milk.

These detergents contain surfactants mixed with fats (oils) that do not produce foam and therefore result very gentle while cleaning effectively.

Due to the presence of fats, they have an emollient and moisturising action and often do not leave a feeling of clean skin (even if rinsed). After a short time, the skin may appear shiny and greasy.

Tip: use only during particularly aggressive anti-acne treatments presenting dryness and irritation of the skin (e.g. topical and systemic treatment with retinoids, chemical peels) or in case of very sensitive skin.

Cleansing milks (No rinse)

These are mixtures of fats without emulsifiers (surfactants) that cannot be rinsed. They can be removed with cotton or a wipe. However, a residual layer of fatty substances on the surface of the skin remains. This layer leaves the skin hydrated but slightly greasy and shiny, which may contribute to the formation of new comedones.

Tip: to be avoided.

Toners and astringents

They may be alcoholic and non-alcoholic. Fortunately, the first ones, which are degreasing and irritating, are no longer used.

The non-alcoholic tonics are aqueous solutions containing vegetable extracts with a soothing and astringent or decongestant action, sometimes containing small amounts of surfactants.

They are usually recommended and used for cleaning the skin or combined with a cleansing milk (No rinse) to remove any residue.

Tip: they are not that helpful and leave a residual surfactants or hydrating substances that could irritate and encourage the formation of new comedones.

Tip: useless and ineffective.

Micellar waters

They are similar to toners. These are aqueous solutions containing plant extracts, emollients and surfactants which, in theory, would have the function of gently cleansing oily or sensitive acneic skin without having to rinse after use. However, they do not cleanse in an appropriate way and surfactants and emollients remain on the skin, which will have a counter-productive action on acne.

Tip: to be avoided. If you have sensitive skin, I would advise to use a rinse-off cleansing milk.

Cleaning masks for oily skin

They often say they have effects of deep cleansing but they actually act in a bland and superficial way.

There are three types:
1.   powder
2.   paste
3.   gel

The first two types are similar. In the first case, the powder is mixed with an aqueous solution so as to prepare a paste (powder in water).

The masks in the form of paste are already-made.

The powders used are generally constituted by zinc oxide with an astringent and soothing action, bentonite and Kaolin with absorbing action, or clay or mud which may contain sulphur (with a keratolytic action: exfoliating and desiccant).

The aqueous solution can vary, based on plant extracts, milk or yoghurt.

A uniform layer is applied to the skin for 20-30 minutes and it is later removed with water. The aqueous component, due to the skin temperature, evaporates causing a decongestant effect and a feeling of freshness. The powders, in addition to any specific chemical action, perform a mechanical adsorbing action on sebum and cellular debris on the surface, leaving the skin cleaner, drier and smoother.

Gel masks are made from polyvinyl alcohol. They can contain astringent, decongesting or exfoliating plant-based active principles. When applied to the skin, they form a transparent thin film which gradually dries out and that can be removed after about 20 minutes.

Even gel masks give a feeling of freshness during application and, after their removal, leave the skin smooth clean and moisturised as an effect of occlusion and reduction of the water evaporation from the epidermis.

Tip: some masks can be helpful when used periodically.

Cleansing or make-up removal wipes

These are wipes moistened or impregnated with an aqueous solution containing emollients and surfactants. They are generally used to remove make-up, but people often erroneously use them to replace the facial cleanser so they do not rinse their face after use, leaving residues of surfactants and emollients that can irritate acne-prone skin.

Tip: to be avoided.

Exfoliants

Exfoliating cleansers in liquid or gel form contain exfoliating ingredients (see next page) in different concentrations that help remove or prevent clogging of the pores.

Tip: they can be effective as part of a carefully balanced acne treatment. They may cause irritation.

Scrubs

The scrubs are cleansers or creamy emulsions containing solid particles of different nature, vegetable or mineral, which typically perform a gentle abrasive action. It is essentially a physical type peeling with a smoothing effect: the dead skin cells are removed and the skin appears smoother and brighter.

However, the action of these solid particles can also cause lesions to the skin, like many small microscopic scratches that can make it very sensitive and irritable, inflame it, or allow the implantation of bacteria and the possibility of infections.

So, how can you get benefits and avoid irritation from scrubs?

- choose a gentle product, with very small particles
- apply to wet skin with slow circular movements and without exerting excessive pressure
- rinse thoroughly with water
- wash your skin with a gentle low-foaming cleanser with mildly acidic pH to restore the acid balance of the skin that prevents the germination of bacteria
- particularly in the presence of active acne, apply a small amount of antibiotic gel on the treated area.

Tip: you can use them regularly on oily, acneic and non sensitive skin.

Exfoliants

Exfoliants such as alpha hydroxy acids (glycolic acid and other fruit acids: malic acid, mandelic acid, etc.) and beta hydroxy acids (like salicylic acid) can be found in cleansers, lotions, creams, serums and gels.

Among exfoliants, there are also retinaldehyde (and retinoids), derivatives of retinol or vitamin A.

They represent one of the cornerstones of anti-acne therapies and treatments.

These substances (such as retinoids, which are classified as drugs and therefore absent in normal cosmetics) act according to different mechanisms, but have exfoliation as a final result, i.e. removing dead cells of the stratum corneum, which occurs in the form of very slight flaking during home treatments.

It is important to stress that this state of mild dryness and flaking generally lasts for a few days or weeks, just the time for your skin to get used to the treatment.

Provoking exfoliation means accelerating the turnover of skin cells. The epidermal turnover normally occurs every 28 days. With exfoliation, instead, you will get it within a smaller number of days: the visible result will be a brighter, smoother and rosier skin. In short, you will have a fresher and cleaner face.

In order to get the best anti-acne results, exfoliation should be mild and performed regularly!

The regular use of exfoliating cosmetics or drugs:

- maintains an accelerated pace of your skin renewal
- maintains or normalises skin structure
- avoids or eliminates the accumulation of pigment and spots
- stimulates the production of new collagen and elastic fibres and hyaluronic acid: this can result in an improvement of the skin weft and scarring (if any)
- improves the absorption, action and the effectiveness of other cosmetic treatments
- well prepares your skin to exfoliating outpatient treatments

In fact, as we will see later on, faster and deeper benefits can be combined to periodic outpatient sessions of peeling and fractional radiofrequency.

Moisturisers

They are oil in water emulsions (lighter and more evanescent) or water in oil (richer and denser).

In my experience, any moisturiser, which causes swelling of the skin cells, worsens the occlusion of the pilosebaceous follicles and neutralises the benefit of exfoliating treatments.

Tip: to be avoided.

Mattifiers

They are oil in water creams, serums, and gels with silica or methacrylates which have matting action (matte effect). In some cases, they also absorb the excess sebum, further reducing the unappealing shiny appearance of oily skin.

They do not have a sebum normalising action, i.e. they do not reduce sebum secretion.

If transparent, even the powder preparations (zinc oxide, titanium dioxide, kaolin, talc and magnesium carbonate, coloured pigments) i.e. face powders have an excellent mattifying action.

Tip: use powder products to avoid the moisturising effect.

Cover creams or make-up products or camouflage creams

In the Moisturisers section, I stated that they worsen or contribute to the clogging of pores and the formation of comedones. As we will see later, even the coloured make-up creams or foundations inevitably have a moisturising action and should be avoided.

In the most practical part of the book, we will later see that people often make the mistake of masking pimples with foundations and stick concealers, which are rich in waxes and fats.

Fortunately, there are also make-up products in the form of compact foundation: they are creams where the powder component (zinc oxide, titanium dioxide, kaolin, talc and magnesium carbonate, coloured pigments) is so predominant that the cream is compact and solid, the moisturising effect is minimised, and there is often a pleasant mattifying, covering and uniforming effect.

Tip: use compact foundations.

TOPICAL DRUGS

In mild cases of acne, the therapy may be merely topical. The anti-acne products for local use are applied on the skin surface at least once a day.

There are mixtures that contain many associated active ingredients, which generally have greater effectiveness. According to their active ingredients and relevant action, we can classify 3 large groups of topical drugs.

ANTISEPTICS

Chlorhexidine

Chlorhexidine has an antiseptic action with a broad spectrum of activity towards gram-positive and gram-negative bacteria, and fungi. It has a bactericidal and fungicidal type of action.

Chlorhexidine is generally used for cleansing skin and pre-surgical cleansing.

For acne, it is available in cleansers and creams.

Since it is a powerful antiseptic with broad spectrum, it kills Propionibacterium acnes as well as other bacteria that usually reside on the skin and are in competition with PA itself. This causes an imbalance in the normal bacterial and fungal flora, which often leads to a worsening of pimples.

It also often causes dryness (and sometimes skin irritation) which leads to a rebound effect with increased production of sebum.

With 2% concentration, it can cause severe and permanent lesions in case of prolonged contact with eyes.

Other side effects may be hypersensitivity and allergic reactions, dermatitis.

Benzoyl peroxide

As the name suggests, it contains peroxide, a highly oxidizing substance which liberates oxygen and kills bacteria including Propionibacterium acnes.

It also has exfoliating and comedolytic effect that contributes to its anti-acne effectiveness.

It may cause irritation, contact dermatitis and increase skin sensitivity to sunlight.

It is available in cleansers, creams and gels.

Micronized Silver - Zinc acetate - Lauric acid

Products containing lauric acid, zinc acetate and micronized silver have proven to be effective on PA strains which have become resistant to antibiotics.

Zinc acetate has:
- a sebostatic action as it inhibits the activity of 5-alpha-reductase type I (an enzyme that converts testosterone into its active form: dihydrotestosterone) at the level of the pilosebaceous follicle
- a bacteriostatic action on PA
- an anti-inflammatory action (reduces the effect of PA on white blood cells which then form pus),
- an antioxidant action

Lauric acid is a fatty acid of plant origin with a very powerful antibacterial action on PA.

Micronized silver has a significant antimicrobial effect: it causes the formation of microscopic holes in the bacterial cell wall.

ANTIBIOTICS

When it comes to acne, antibiotics (both applied locally and orally administered) are used for the antibacterial action on PA but in particular for their anti-inflammatory action.

In fact, if you reduce PA, you also reduce the action of bacterial lipase (enzymes produced by PA) on sebum and thus a decrease of free fatty acids. Remember that these are oxidised with the consequent formation of the inflammatory free radicals within the pilosebaceous follicle and skin surface.

Moreover, they reduce the effect of PA on white blood cells with a reduction of pus formation and its destructive action on dermis.

The antibiotics applied locally inhibit the growth of Propionibacterium acnes and are only effective when acne is inflamed – only on pimples, not on comedones.

However, their prolonged use (about three months) often causes the appearance of resistant bacteria, although this seems a reversible phenomenon. For this reason, it is advisable to suspend antibiotic therapy (so it does not become ineffective) and replace it with an alternative antibacterial product for a given period of time.

Clindamycin phosphate

It has very effective bacteriostatic action.
It is available in gel and lotion form with 1% concentration.

Erythromycin

It is part of macrolide antibiotics with bacteriostatic action.
It is available in gel, cream and lotion form with 3% concentration.

Fusidic acid

The drug acts on gram-positive cocci, staphylococci (including penicillin-resistant strains), streptococci and pneumococci. It is mainly used in pyoderma but is also effective in acne.

Meclocycline sulphosalicylate

This is a tetracycline with a bacteriostatic action. It is available in cream form.

HORMONES

Spironolactone

This has an anti-androgen action and is available in cream form. It is contraindicated for men. It should reduce the activity of the sebaceous glands and then act on the excessive production of sebum, but it is very inefficient in practice.

TOPICAL RETINOIDS

Retinoic acid or tretinoin

Tretinoin is a real anti-acne drug which has revealed to be remarkably effective in fighting pimples.

Tretinoin is a retinoid, which is a derivative of vitamin A, used for many years in acne treatments in gel, cream and lotion form.

It is very powerful and its effects are both superficial and deep.

You can see the benefits for acne after about 3 months. At an early stage, you may experience a temporary worsening of the skin because of the irritation and inflammation of comedones upon which it acts.

At the skin surface level, it acts by accelerating the replacement of epidermal cells, causing a continuous (very light, almost invisible) exfoliation, which removes the horny plugs of blackheads and whiteheads, and reduces their formation, preventing the appearance of new pimples.

As for all medications and remedies for acne, you should not rely on hearsay, but be followed by a dermatologist who will assess if tretinoin is really suitable for your skin type and acne.

The microexfoliation looks like a mild state of dryness of the skin, which, at times, is more intense and accompanied by redness, itching and irritation: here comes the so-called "retinoid dermatitis", the most frequent side effect when you have a very sensitive skin or when you have applied it too much. In this case, you should contact the dermatologist who prescribed the treatment and, probably, suspend the anti-acne treatment for a few days in order to give time to our skin to recover its balance.

The deep effects related to skin aging occur gradually in the dermis: after about 6 months of regular use of tretinoin, the damage caused by the sun (photoaging) are greatly reduced, the amount of new collagen and hyaluronic acid content increases and the skin appears smoother, bright and robust, with a visible and progressive decrease of fine wrinkles.

For its anti-wrinkle action, tretinoin has been ranked among cosmeceuticals, which are active ingredients with a cosmetic and pharmacological action.

Isotretinoin

This is a very powerful molecule, similar to tretinoin but less effective and more irritating – in my experience.

It is available in cream or gel form.

It is also used in tablets for general route, as we will see shortly.

Adapalene

This is another retinoid, which is also available in cream or gel form.

In addition to having the effects of other retinoids (i.e. eliminate blackheads and whiteheads and slow down or prevent their formation), it has fewer irritating effects. It actually has a real anti-inflammatory activity as it inhibits lipoxygenase, the enzyme which causes the formation of free radicals from the free fatty acids of the sebum.

Retinaldehyde

This is a natural derivative of vitamin A or retinol: in fact, it also forms within cells, where it builds a natural reserve of retinoids which then act on DNA by accelerating cell renewal and preventing pores clogging. This prevents precisely that stratification which clogs pores.

It is not a drug, it is found in cosmetic creams often combined with alpha-hydroxy acids.

It rarely causes irritation.

NICOTINAMIDE or niacinamide or vitamin B3 or vitamin PP

In 1995, a clinical study (Int J Dermatol. 1995) carried out by Shalita AR, 76 patients with moderately severe acne were divided into two groups and treated with nicotinamide gel at 4% and clindamycin gel at 1% over a period of two months. The benefits in the two groups apparently seemed to be overlapping or similar, but there was no control group following a placebo treatment. For this reason, the results should be considered controversial or scarcely significant.

SYSTEMIC DRUGS

Systemic drugs are generally administered orally in cases of very inflamed or severe acne: pustular and nodulocystic acne. In any case, they are prescribed when local therapies are not enough to put pimples under control.

ANTIBIOTICS

In acne, the systemic antibiotic therapy is based on the same antibiotics that we have seen in topical therapy: **tetracyclines, macrolides** and **clindamycin** (more rarely).

Even systemic antibiotics are used to reduce the population of Propionibacterium acnes and counteract its contribution to acne inflammation.

In recent years, the knowledge on the pathogenesis of acne has expanded and more importance is being given to comedolytic and exfoliating agents – and so it should be.

For this reason, systemic antibiotic therapies should be used properly and for short periods:

- to avoid side effects;
- to avoid the occurrence of bacterial resistance (unfortunately, ever more frequent) that make them ineffective towards others germs which are far more dangerous;
- because they are useless in the long term, if the local therapy is carried out well.

HORMONES

Oestro-progestogens

Oestro-progestogens are drugs that contain, in adequate proportion, oestrogen and progesterone, the female sex hormones.

In other words, oestro-progestones mixtures correspond to the "birth control pill": they simulate a pregnancy and put ovaries at rest, blocking their production of female and male sex hormones.

What is important is that there is no ovarian production of male hormones (testosterone, etc.), which affect the increased production of sebum and formation of pimples.

The pill is needed when there are specific hormonal disorders:

- the levels of male hormones (androgens) in the blood are above normal
- there are ovarian microcysts or cysts (polycystic ovary verified by transvaginal ultrasound performed by the gynaecologist) that lead to a greater production of male hormones by the ovaries.

Even when hormone levels are normal, the pill can still be useful in women when it is suspected that androgen receptors located in the sebaceous glands and pilosebaceous follicles are more sensitive: the sebaceous glands are more stimulated to produce sebum.

The degree of hormone receptor sensitivity is genetically influenced, so there is a family and hereditary predisposition.

Anti-androgens: cyproterone acetate

The anti-androgens are drugs that counteract the action of androgen hormones by blocking their peripheral receptors.

The most used is the cyproterone acetate. It can (and should) be combined with the pill as a separate medication or it may be present in the same product in combination with oestro-progestogens. The anti-androgens are particularly suitable when, in addition to acne, there are signs of hirsutism (excessive hair growth, hair loss)

It is needless to say these hormonal therapies with oestro-progestogens and anti-androgens are for women only.

RETINOIDS: Isotretinoin

Isotretinoin is a retinoid, derivative of vitamin A, and is the most effective oral anti-acne medication. It is prescribed by a dermatologist only for severe and resistant forms of acne as it can have serious side effects.

In fact, it is necessary to do specific lab tests before and during treatment and undergo regular dermatological check-ups.

It has a powerful action on keratinocytes (skin cells) and many other cells as it acts on cellular DNA.

Isotretinoin is a highly teratogenic drug: it causes serious birth defects in pregnant patients.

For this reason, in the rare cases where it is necessary to prescribe isotretinoin to a female patient, the doctor must combine it with an effective and prolonged birth control therapy.

Isotretinoin acts on all the factors that cause pimples. The positive effects of isotretinoin include:

1. reduction of the sebaceous glands size and sebaceous secretion
2. consequent reduction of the bacteria present in the pilosebaceous follicle contributing to acne inflammation
3. thickness reduction of the stratum corneum (the outermost layer of the epidermis, consisting of dead cells) with reduction of pores occlusion and formation of blackheads and whiteheads.

It is generally administered for about 4-5-6 months and the cycle can be possibly repeated in case the acne reappears.

The side effects of isotretinoin already begin to show up during the first month. However, they are considered "normal" as they frequently remain until the end of the therapy.

The patient may experience:
-   extremely dry skin that often becomes red, with burning sensation or itching
-   dry eyes and mucous membranes
-   occasional small nosebleeds
-   photosensitivity

The side effects of isotretinoin which are NOT considered normal and should suggest its immediate suspension are:

- an increase in triglycerides and cholesterol (to be kept under regular control)
- an increase in blood sugar
- headache
- worsening of acne with formation of hypertrophic scars
- hepatitis, pancreatitis
- depression

In some cases you may experience an intense and widespread worsening of your acne: pimples become deeper, more inflamed and painful.

Sometimes this is due to a low dose (under-dosing) of the drug that, paradoxically, only further "stimulates" and inflame pimples.

In conclusion, as I tell my patients, isotretinoin is the most extreme treatment for acne. Since it is a real "atomic bomb" for pimples and body, it should be used only when no other home or outpatient care (e.g. chemical peel) has worked.

HERBAL MEDICINE

There are several natural remedies for acne; some of them are effective, some of them are not.

They have been recently rediscovered for various reasons:

- when possible, natural and gentle remedies are preferred
- antibiotics often cause the appearance of resistant bacteria which are difficult to eradicate.

Nevertheless, in case of acne or any other pathology, you should bear in mind that herbal medicine always represents a complementary therapy to conventional medical therapy.

This does not mean that it does not provide benefits. It can help prepare the overall organism and skin to more effective treatments, especially during the maintenance phase, when acne is stabilised and kept under control also by measures and habits of a healthy lifestyle.

Let us examine the herbs that can help you in fighting pimples. Some of them were enhanced by very recent scientific and clinical research and used in the form of dermocosmetic products or food supplements. In any case, it is always possible to use them in the form of infusions, decoctions and hydroalcoholic tinctures, i.e. the typical herbal preparations.

Echinacea

This strengthens the immune system, the activity of white blood cells in particular.

It can be helpful in fighting bacterial, viral and fungal infections in general: it can indeed be recommended in winter as a supplement to help prevent flu and respiratory tract infections.

This has proved to be useful also in contrasting the inflammatory action of Propionibacterium acnes.

Furthermore, it also seems that echinacea promotes tissue repair, which is useful in fighting acne and acne marks such as blemishes and scars: reducing inflammation and stimulating skin healing, ensures a quicker improvement of pimples and a reduction of their depth.

Thyme

The virtues of thyme have been well-known for years: the essential oil of thyme has antiseptic properties useful for respiratory, intestinal, and skin infections.

In some cosmetics, in cream or powder form, this activity is already used but only for deodorant purpose.

A recent study conducted in the laboratories of Leeds Metropolitan University found out that the most effective natural remedy for pimples is precisely the thyme tincture.

The researchers then showed a good antibacterial ability of thyme tincture against Propionibacterium acnes.

We already knew the antiseptic and purifying properties of thyme and other herbal ingredients such as marigold and myrrh tincture, but this study clearly showed these actions on the acne bacterium.

What is even more relevant in the carried out study is the comparison with other anti-acne antibiotics and benzoyl peroxide, a very effective antiseptic substance used for treating pimples.

Yet it seems that the effectiveness of the antibacterial activity of thyme tincture against the Propionibacterium acnes is equal to antibiotics and slightly higher than benzoyl peroxide: it kills PA in just five minutes of exposure.

This opens up new possibilities in the treatment of acne, especially in its mild forms. Thyme extracts can be added into cosmetic products such as cleansers, anti-acne creams and gels: they would become effective, gentle and pleasant without causing side effects such as irritation and allergies.

Burdock

The root of this plant seems to have purifying and microbicidal properties (on gram-positive bacteria such as staphylococci and streptcocci) that might be helpful also for treating acne.

Dandelion

The root of this plant are used for preparing decoctions and alcoholic tinctures for detoxifying purpose. It contains phytosterols and tannins. It stimulates the liver and biliary function and has a mild laxative action.

Serenoa repens

It is a plant rich in saturated and unsaturated fatty acids and phytosterols. It has inhibitory action on 5-alpha-reductase, the enzyme that converts testosterone (T) into dihydrotestosterone (DHT), which stimulates the secretion of sebum.

FOOD SUPPLEMENTS AND NUTRACEUTICALS

Food supplements are concentrated sources of nutrients that supplement your normal diet with the purpose of promoting body functions and improving its health.

They can only be used orally and they are not drugs that treat diseases or dietary products for losing weight.

There are commercially available in various forms: capsules, tablets, powder preparations, drops, syrups.

According to their ingredients, there are different types of food supplements. Let us examine the main ones and the ones that may be more useful to treat acne.

SUPPLEMENTS BASED ON HERBS OR DERIVATIVES

In acne, it might be useful to take food supplements containing the herbs mentioned earlier.

Serenoa repens

This comes from the berries of a palm tree. It has a bland antiandrogenic effect, primarily through a direct action on the dihydrotestosterone receptors but also through indirect action i.e. inhibiting the 5-alpha-reductase enzyme, which is present at the level of the pilosebaceous follicles and transforms the testosterone into dihydrotestosterone.

It is found in supplements used in the treatment of androgenic alopecia or common baldness and prostate hypertrophy. In acne, it may have a mild sebum normalising effect.

VITAMIN SUPPLEMENTS

Vitamins are essential substances for your health and proper body functioning: they intervene in metabolic processes and enzymatic reactions.

Most vitamins are not synthesised by your body and should therefore be introduced with food.

A lack of vitamins, often due to a wrong diet, or an increase in intake may cause mild or severe ailments.

Some vitamins are useful in treating acne and some are not. For example, if group B vitamins, which are abundantly found in yeast that is often mistakenly used for the treatment of pimples, are taken in excess, they can cause worsening or onset of acne (vitamin B acne)

Here are all the vitamins that can have beneficial effects on acne.

Vitamin E or tocopherol
It is a lipophilic molecule (high affinity with lipids) with a remarkable antioxidant action: it protects polyunsaturated fatty acids that are part of cell membranes and sebum against free radicals.

At the level of the skin, it then counteracts the inflammation and the formation of comedones

Vitamin C or ascorbic acid
It is a hydrophilic vitamin (high affinity with water) with antioxidant and anti-inflammatory action at the level of cells and tissues.

Nicotinamide or niacinamide or vitamin B3 or vitamin PP
The benefits of nicotinamide via oral or local application in acne are very controversial. In theory, the vitamin should play an anti-inflammatory action but the administration as a food supplement can lead to side effects such as flushing (sudden reddening of the face), heartburn, itching, headache and chronic liver disease.

In my experience, I have not seen visible benefits neither via local treatment nor via oral administration.

Inositol, or vitamin B7
Inositol is an essential substance for the body, which is perfectly able of producing it on its own. It is can be found in many foods.

The richest food sources of inositol are bran, whole grains, wheat germs, brewer's yeast, legumes (beans), citrus fruits and meats in general, liver in particular.

In fact, it is precisely produced at the level of liver and kidney – the latter also has the task to eliminate any excess. It is a water-soluble substance that does not accumulate in the body. Indeed, as a supplement, it is well tolerated and devoid of toxicity.

The myo-inositol, the active form, is a molecule similar to glucose; it is in fact an alcoholic sugar.

It has an important metabolic activity control of fats and sugars and is involved in the insulin production. In cases of insulin resistance or type II diabetes, inositol has showed the ability to improve the overall metabolism and counteract a possible increase in blood sugar and insulin.

It is essential for hair growth and preventing baldness.

It has a general detoxifying action, on the liver in particular.

Inositol and polycystic ovary syndrome (PCOS)

The myo-inositol and D-chiro-inositol have a positive effect on ovarian function and lead to a reduction of:

- LH
- testosterone
- prolactin
- LH/FSH ratio
- triglycerides
- insulin

Moreover, myo-inositol also helps restore a regular menstrual cycle with ovulation: 50% of female patients already begin to ovulate after one month. In the 70-80% of cases, it restores the menstrual cycle in about 60 days.

In a study (published in the Gynecological Endocrinology magazine) carried out on 50 women (average age of 25 years) suffering from PCOS with acne and hirsutism, after 6 months of treatment with myo-inositol and folic acid, a significant reduction of androstenedione and testosterone was shown, with consequent improvement of acne (in 53% of cases) and hirsutism.

In another study, it was shown that after only 6-8 weeks, the combination of 4 g of myo-inositol with 400 mg of folic acid improved insulin sensitivity and reduced the circulating levels of triglycerides.

However, for those who suffer from acne and polycystic ovary, introducing inositol with food is not enough; food supplements are necessary.

Inositol and stress

Since it is part of phospholipids, its biological role also includes control activities of the nervous system cell function with anxiolytic and antidepressant action.

Clinical studies results have shown that inositol has an anxiolytic power similar to that of benzodiazepines: so it can act as a tranquilliser without any side effects and be effective against insomnia.

As part of acne therapy, inositol can be used as a vitamin supplement for its many beneficial balancing effects on fats and sugars metabolism and hormonal levels, its overall detoxifying action and its anxiolytic and antidepressant action.

The recommended dose is 2 g a day, usually combined with folic acid.

ANTIOXIDANT SUPPLEMENTS
Vitamin E and C also belong to this category.

Alpha-lipoic acid
It is a powerful antioxidant at the level of both extracellular fluid and cell membranes as it is soluble in both water and fats.

As all antioxidants, it has a potential anti-inflammatory action also on acne.

Dermocosmetic products in cream containing alpha-lipoic acid are mainly used for anti-aging purpose. Some creams are also prescribed for anti-acne therapies, but (in my experience) they are little or non-effective because the pro-acneic moisturising effect overcomes the benefits of a possible anti-inflammatory action.

Its antioxidant action could instead be more useful and effective as a supplement in tablets.

Green tea polyphenols
Among green tea polyphenols, catechins have a powerful antioxidant, anticancer and anti-inflammatory action. According to some studies, they seem to inhibit the activity of 5-alpha-reductase, an enzyme which converts testosterone into dihydrotestosterone.

Green tea may therefore help to normalise sebum secretion and acne inflammation. In any case, the studies on its properties are conflicting.

Moreover, green tea contains theanine, an amino acid that is rapidly absorbed by the intestine and distributed to tissues. It rapidly overcomes the blood-brain barrier by increasing the levels of GABA, a neurotransmitter upon which many anxiolytics and sedative drugs also act upon.

The soothing effect of theanine seems to partially contrast the excitatory properties of the caffeine found in green tea: at higher concentrations, the final result seems to be a feeling of wellbeing and calm.

MINERAL SUPPLEMENTS

Minerals or trace elements such as magnesium and potassium are inorganic substances present in our body which are part of various physiological and biochemical processes. They are essential for our body's balance and vital functions.

Like vitamins, our body is unable to produce them so they are introduced with food. We eliminate them via sweat and urine.

Magnesium chloride

Our body contains about 25 grams of magnesium. It is mainly found in bones, muscles, brain and other organs.

Magnesium is necessary for an adequate assimilation of calcium and potassium, the correct and efficient functioning of many enzymes, the production of energy by cells, and the functioning of vitamins (e.g. vitamin C is only active in the presence of magnesium ions).

Magnesium is an essential nutrient: our body constantly consumes it and in order to maintain an adequate level in body tissues, it needs to be taken regularly with food.

In case of minor deficiencies, many mild disorders are likely to occur: anxiety, mild depression, cardiac arrhythmias, fatigue, weakness and muscle spasms (cramps), irritability and insomnia, constipation, PMS.

It is an essential constituent of chlorophyll, the green pigment fundamental for the life of plants. And it is well known that chlorophyll has a deodorising, bacteriostatic, healing and tonic action – probably due to the presence of magnesium.

The RDA (recommended daily allowance) of magnesium is 360 mg a day for a 60 kg woman and 420 mg a day for a 70 kg man. It has been used for a long time as magnesium oxide in antacids drugs and as magnesium hydroxide and sulphate in laxatives.

The crystallised magnesium chloride is mainly extracted from seawater and has a bitter taste.

Magnesium chloride is used as a food supplement because it is an organic salt easier to assimilate.

It can be used in powder diluted in water or in tablets.

It seems to have a:

- detoxifying
- calming and balancing
- bacteriostatic
- potentiating (on white blood cells) and
- energising action.

For these global actions, magnesium chloride may be also useful as a food supplement for acne, if considered appropriate by the dermatologist.

AMINO ACID SUPPLEMENTS

Amino acids are the molecules that form proteins and peptides: they are also needed for the synthesis of hormones and neurotransmitters – substances that allow cells communicate with each other.

Tryptophan

It is an amino acid precursor of serotonin, the neurotransmitter of good mood and serenity. Tryptophan allows the formation of melatonin, the hormone which is the basis of the sleep-wake rhythm.

Supplements made from tryptophan and melatonin are very useful during stressful times, when you need a rebalance.

FATTY ACID SUPPLEMENTS

As previously mentioned, fatty acids are divided into saturated fatty acids (the "bad ones) and unsaturated fatty acids (the "good" ones). Unsaturated fatty acids have a key role in the adequate development of many metabolic and biological functions of our body

Fish oil

It is often synonymous of Omega 3 as it is the richest animal source. Once again, omega-3s have multiple functions, among which the antioxidant and anti-inflammatory function, the main ones.

Supplementing your diet with fish oil, i.e. omega-3, is helpful to make sebum and skin cell membranes less "attackable" by free radicals, which means reducing comedogenesis and acne inflammation.

The usual recommended dose is 2 g a day.

Chia seeds or salvia hispanica

They contain many amino acids and are particularly rich in sulfur amino acids such as methionine and cysteine, which are essential for the formation of the keratin of skin's stratum corneum and cutaneous attachments (hair and nails).

They also contain significant amounts of flavonoids, vitamins and essential fatty acids (especially omega 3, such as alpha-linoleic) that confer antioxidant and anti-inflammatory properties.

Moreover, they are rich in fibres which, with their ability to absorb water, give a sense of satiety and promote intestinal transit, so they are also useful in low calories and detoxifying diets and in case of glycemic intolerance, diabetes and constipation.

These properties can also be exploited in in diets for acne patients with beneficial effects on body and skin.

Flax seeds

They are rich in fibres (mucilages) with an emollient and soothing action for gastrointestinal mucous membranes and skin. However, what is most important is that they represent the richest vegetable source of omega 3, superior to chia seeds and fish oil.

PROBIOTIC SUPPLEMENTS

In our digestive system there are 100,000 billion bacteria belonging to more than 400 bacterial species (intestinal microflora): they constitute a real ecosystem.

This ecosystem is often damaged or destroyed not only by poor nutrition and junk food but also by factors such as physical and emotional stress, drugs, and infections.

However, the health of gastrointestinal flora is crucial not only for the good functioning of our intestine, but also to strengthen the natural defences of our body against the invasion of bacteria and pathogenic germs through the intestinal wall itself and not only.

Probiotics are microorganisms that have positive effects on the health of the organisms that host them. They are able to go through the gastric barrier and reach the intestine "alive".

They are generally found in natural yoghurt and cheeses but, in order to have significant effects, it is necessary to absorb higher amounts via some yoghurt-based products and specific supplements.

Main functions of probiotics:

- help rebalance the intestinal flora
- normalise intestinal functions by contrasting the onset of infections and intestinal tumours
- have a rather laxative and therefore detoxifying action
- promote the absorption of nutrients
- produce group B vitamins
- reduce intestinal absorption of fats (cholesterol) and sugars

- are crucial to maintaining the efficiency of our immune system

In recent years, researchers have observed that orally ingested lactobacilli can stimulate the activity of immune cells, which detect and kill cancer cells and invading microorganisms.

According to recent studies, the antimicrobial action of Acidophilus is due to the production of:
- lactic acid (which reduces the intestinal pH)
- hydrogen peroxide
- antibiotic substances.

In particular, Acidophilus DDS-1 produces remarkable amounts of acidophiline, the most powerful natural antibiotic.

Many of the benefits of Bifidus supplementation are generally similar to those of Acidophilus, although with particular reference to the large intestine where Bifidus mostly implants.

The administration of bifidobacteria, especially if combined with synergistic fibres and herbs, can also solve serious constipation problems and improve the intestinal and liver function.

Supplements and yoghurts containing lactobacilli and/or living bifidobacteria may be beneficial in skin diseases such as acne and rosacea precisely because they would act on the intestine-nervous system-skin axis.

Impacts on acne and skin infections

Various studies have shown the connection between intestinal flora alteration and the appearance of skin conditions. This has led to the intuition of the use of probiotics in the treatment of pimples.

More than 70 years ago, Stokes and Pillsbury hypothesised a close connection between the nervous system, intestine and skin, and thus between emotional states, changes in intestinal microflora, and skin inflammatory processes such as acne, rosacea, and seborrheic dermatitis.

In the late 1964, Dr Robert Siver (Journal of Medical Society of New Jersey) treated 300 cases of youth acne via administration of Acidophilus and Bulgaricus, obtaining an improvement in the clinical picture in 80% of cases.

Some international studies have shown a correlation between oral administration of probiotics and an improvement of acne.

A recent Korean research on 56 patients with acne found that daily administration of products containing living Lactobacillus reduced the number of acne lesions and sebum production in 12 weeks.

In an Italian study, half of the patients were given probiotic supplements along with a traditional therapy for acne or rosacea. The other half of patients, instead, followed standard therapies only. The group that had also taken probiotic-based supplements experienced a more pronounced improvement in acne and rosacea lesions.

Another recent Italian study has also evaluated the effects of the administration of a Lactobacillus rhamnosus T12 supplement in patients with seborrheic acne and seborrheic dermatitis. After only 1 month, there was a reduction of surface sebum and normalisation of skin pH, with slight improvement in acne.

Lactobacillus rhamnosus T12 has an immune-modulating action; it seemingly modulates skin inflammation and this may explain its beneficial effects on acne.

Certainly, the actions of probiotics may explain why they are helpful for patients with acne, especially in those cases where the following actions are needed:

- detoxifying
- supporting an anti-acne antibiotic therapy
- supporting a systemic retinoid therapy
- integrating a low calorie or low glycemic index diet combined with anti-acne therapies.

As I will explain later, in order to combat the acne and rosacea inflammatory processes linked to the intestine-nervous system-skin axis, it would be useful to:
- manage and reduce stress
- adjust your diet
- introduce lactobacilli and bifidobacteria via oral administration

Probiotics would strengthen and enrich microflora, creating a healthy barrier and preventing the production of toxins and inflammation that contribute to the worsening of acne (and rosacea).

There are some cosmetics formulas (creams, masks or cleansers) which include probiotics.

They may perform a protective action:

in acne and rosacea, the microorganisms present in the skin are attacked by the immune system through an inflammatory process which leads to erythema, papules and pustules.

Locally applied probiotics interfere by "distracting" immune system cells present in the skin, which would then react less against the bacteria and parasites involved in acne and rosacea.

They may also have an antimicrobial action as they produce natural antibiotics.

Many patients, with acne or with healthy skin, have tried the application of home-made yoghurt masks in an attempt to improve their appearance and condition, but there is no evidence of the effectiveness of these remedies.

Adding yoghurt to your diet or supplementing it with oral probiotics can surely benefit the body in general, but it cannot be considered an exclusive treatment for acne or rosacea.

It can be a complementary therapy that integrates and strengthens the anti-acne diet and treatment, helping reduce the degree of skin inflammation.

FIBRE SUPPLEMENTS

Fibres are part of plant foods that the body does not assimilate. They are not degraded by gastrointestinal tract enzymes. They perform important mechanical and metabolic functions that can also affect the intestinal bacterial flora. They are present in fruit, vegetables, cereals and seeds.

They help improve intestinal regularity and reduce fat absorption.

In acne, they may be useful when a low calorie and low glycemic index diet is needed (at the intestinal level, they bind glucose by slowing down its absorption and reducing blood pressure), to rebalance the intestinal bacterial flora (see probiotics) and for their depurative action.

Oat bran

Oat bran is a food rich in fibres (20%), essentially soluble fibres and pectin, and mineral salts such as magnesium, potassium, zinc, copper and manganese.

It also contains folic acid, vitamin A, C, E and group B vitamins. The soluble fibres bind to a large amount of water (from twenty to forty times their weight) and therefore they swell inside the stomach giving an immediate sense of satiety.

Even more interesting is that soluble oat bran fibres are beta-glucans. These are molecules with high-strength antioxidant properties, with a soothing and anti-inflammatory effect at the intestine level. Moreover, as we have seen in the paragraph dedicated to probiotics, this has a beneficial effect on the intestine-nervous system-skin axis.

Actions:
- reducing cholesterol levels
- reducing sugar absorption and stabilising blood sugar
- promoting the growth of intestinal bacterial flora that feeds on the soluble fibres contained therein
- providing a sense of satiety, weight loss
- soothing and softening intestinal walls and protecting them from inflammation
- promoting bowel peristalsis by contrasting constipation

Oat bran has been recently re-evaluated in low calorie and detoxifying diets due to its numerous and remarkable effects.

We recommend a daily consumption of about 40 g a day (about 2-3 tablespoons) to be added to yoghurt, milk or vegetable soups.

To be avoided in cases of gastro-intestinal disorders, celiac disease, irritable colon, abdominal swelling and nickel allergies (as oat bran contains a fair amount of nickel).

Like any other fibre, its excessive consumption may reduce the intestinal absorption of vitamins and minerals.

Psyllium seeds
They contain high levels of highly hydrophilic fibres (mucilages) that bind to large amounts of water by swelling and forming a gel.

If introduced with food, they swell in the stomach giving a sense of satiety (so they are frequently used in weight loss diets) and then get into the intestine where they facilitate and regulate bowel emptying.

The Psyllium mucilages have a softening, soothing and anti-inflammatory action on the gastrointestinal mucous membranes: they therefore serve to counteract constipation and balance the intestinal function.

OUTPATIENT TREATMENTS

Outpatient treatments are medical treatments which, due to their complexity, are to be performed at a dermatological clinic and under the strict control of a specialist.

As I often say to my patients: everyone has the ability to apply an acid onto the skin and perform a chemical peel, but not everyone has the right knowledge experience to choose which acid to use, the type of peeling to perform, understand what is happening to the skin second by second, understand how skin reacts and will react and anticipate and manage the post-treatment course, avoiding side effects and complications.

I need to clarify that, in case of acne, outpatient treatments are not a definitive cure – as many want you to believe. There are no treatments or therapies able to permanently eliminate pimples in a short period of time.

Furthermore, outpatient treatments are not enough to win against acne as acne tends to be persistent and, as we have seen, comedones and pimples formation is a continuous process. It is necessary to constantly fight acne with home treatments, which are crucial and indispensable.

However, outpatient treatments for acne give you great and rapid benefits: they are important, but you should consider them complementary to home treatments.

Their greatest benefit is the speed with which improvements in acne and the depth of skin cleansing are achieved, with progressive removal of comedones.

And a less inflamed and cleaner skin reacts even better to home treatments.

A patient who sees his/her skin rapidly improved becomes more and more confident and motivated to continue the treatment constantly.

This creates a positive cycle that leads to the maintenance of the result: a skin free from pimples.

CHEMICAL PEELING

Chemical peeling is a dermatological treatment that, in Italy, was previously little known to the general public and was carried out by a small number of dermatologists and plastic surgeons.

Since 1993, following the marketing of glycolic acid cosmetics, the chemical peeling technique has widely spread.

Peeling consists in the application of one or more chemicals onto the skin in order to obtain a controlled destruction of skin layers with consequent desquamation (cell replacement acceleration), epidermal regeneration and stimulation of dermal repair with formation of new collagen.

Depending on its depth, we can classify chemical peeling as follows:

- Very superficial
- Superficial
- Medium-depth
- Deep

Clearly, the greater the depth of the peeling, the greater the stimulation and skin repair, the greater the benefits that can be obtained, but the higher the chances of complications.

In the United States, the technique is considered as a surgical act, and therefore of close medical relevance, as it passes through the superficial epidermal layers. However, it is possible for non-medical practitioners to perform very superficial peelings, provided they are under the supervision of a specialist doctor.

In Italy, in spite of the application of the European Directive on cosmetics and their use, which establishes a clear boundary between chemical substances for cosmetic use and those for other uses, regulations appear to be more confusing and this may sometimes favour situations where peeling is carried out by qualified practitioners, non-specialist doctors, non-medical practitioners without any supervision by a specialist doctor.

Very superficial peeling

Very superficial peeling is achieved by applying glycolic acid solutions at concentrations between 50% and 70%, for a variable time depending on the skin type of the patient.

Subjectively, the patient feels a mild sensation of widespread dizziness for a few minutes, the skin becomes erythematosus and after about 3 days a slightly visible desquamation appears and lasts for 5-7 days.

It is indicated to obtain a removal of skin opacity due to a slowing stratum corneum cells turnover, and to attenuate surface pigmentary alterations.

It is often necessary to do multiple sessions in order to get more pronounced results.

The limits are given by its mild, very superficial action, which makes it poorly effective for blemishes such as vulgar acne, scars, wrinkles.

Superficial peeling

Superficial peeling is performed with 70% glycolic acid, 15%-20% trichloroacetic acid, 30% salicylic acid, Jessner solution, Unna's paste (40% resorcinol) or 40% piruvic acid.

In this case, a diffuse burning sensation occurs and a more intense erythema appears; you can observe frosting i.e. a whitening of the skin. The following exfoliation is clearly visible and lasts for 7-10 days.

Superficial peeling is indicated for the treatment of comedonal and papulopustular acne, post-acne superficial scarring, hyperpigmentations such as sun-freckles and melasma, mild photo-aging such as surface roughness of cheeks and periocular areas.

The number and frequency of the sessions can be variable and depends on the blemish and patient's response.

Medium-depth peeling

In medium-depth peelings, specialists can either use 35-41% trichloroacetic acid to perform the so-called combined or mixed peelings (using two or more acids in the same session) or apply only 88% phenol.

In this case, the burning sensation is very intense, which sometimes require a preoperative sedation. In the following hours, edema appears. The post-peeling progress is quite challenging for the patient (it is advisable to postpone any social or work commitments) as the skin becomes dark and after about 5 days a large-scale exfoliation occurs. This fades within 8-10 days.

It is mainly indicated for papulopustular and nodulocystic acne, acne and varicella scarring, epidermal-dermal melasma, and photo-aging with more pronounced wrinkles. It is important to point out that expression or mimic wrinkles and deep scars get little benefit from superficial and medium-depth peels (in this case, the best remedy is to combine intradermal hyaluronic acid systems that fill and also lift wrinkles and deeper scars).

Deep peeling

Deep peeling is rarely used as it is a very complex and challenging technique; it is very painful and requires preoperative sedation and monitoring.

It can be indicated in cases of a marked degree of skin photo-aging with widespread and accentuated wrinkles, and scarring.

In all cases, as far as post-peeling is concerned, total photo-protection is essential in order to prevent the onset of post-inflammatory hyperpigmentation.

Some remarks based on personal experience in treating acne:

Trichloroacetic acid is very useful in outpatient treatments for acne vulgaris: in order to achieve a visible improvement with a marked reduction in inflamed lesions and comedones, 3 to 6 sessions (performed weekly or biweekly) of superficial or medium peeling are usually enough (depending on the overall clinical picture).

When combined with topical home treatments, trichloroacetic acid often does not necessitate the systemic administration of antibiotics.

In some cases of acne and particular types of skin, Glycolic acid (due to its intense moisturising action) may cause worsening in comedones formation and follicular inflammation.

However, it may be useful for treating dry and prematurely aged skin with epidermal patches (on average, 7 to 10 sessions to be carried out every 7-10 days).

Although glycolic acid peeling is often presented by mass media as a fairly simple and risk-free technique, in reality it is not like this: its penetration into the skin may not be uniform and can lead to many complications, including scarring.

Medium-depth peelings make significant improvements on specific cases of nodulocystic acne with scarring: you can often avoid using isotretinoin via oral administration by combining a series of sessions to a local therapy and oral antibiotics.

EXFOLIATING FRACTIONAL RADIOFREQUENCY

Fractional radiofrequency is an innovative technique that has proven to be a viable, less invasive and cheaper alternative to the laser for the treatment of various skin conditions.

During the fractional radiofrequency treatment, the device probe produces an electromagnetic wave able to create an adjustable ablation of superficial skin layers – just as is the case with the light energy of the various types of laser.

Any energy (whether electromagnetic, light or electric) affecting the skin's tissue turns into heat i.e. thermic energy.

This is what is obtained with lasers or with diathermocoagulation in order to necrotise skin lesions.

In the case of fractional radiofrequency, **high temperatures are not reached** and the tissue is not damaged.

While fractional laser reaches temperatures of about 170 degrees which can damage tissue, fractional radiofrequency operates with much lower temperatures (between 50 and 60 degrees) and allow for a greater comfort of treatment (which does not require anaesthesia) and a much faster skin repair.

Microdischarges produce a series of **micro holes** (not visible to the naked eye) whose diameter and depth vary depending on the power, frequency and time of application. What is crucial is that the distance between these micro holes is only a few microns; the skin repair begins exactly from the areas of healthy skin tissue between one hole and another. The repair occurs quickly and optimally, with rapid healing without desquamation and discomfort.

In the case of acne, it is then possible to perform a superficial and smoothing skin exfoliation by **removing the skin's superficial layers**, just as with a chemical peeling but without burning, exfoliation and visible scabs. The skin is smooth and bright due to an immediate micro-vaporisation of the superficial layers, and it may appear mildly dry in the following days, with a micro-desquamation that leads to the removal of horny plugs of open comedones (blackheads) and the expulsion of superficial closed comedones (whiteheads).

During treatment, ozone is also developed, with disinfecting action on pimples and biostimulant for the skin.

With weekly or biweekly sessions, the benefits are progressive: the skin becomes cleaner and cleaner and the number of pimples and comedones is reduced.

In addition, fractional radiofrequency can treat acne scarring, both punctiform and crateriform scars. However, a more visible improvement of deeper scars can be obtained only if other treatments are performed.

Fractional radiofrequency is practically painless and can be performed without outpatient anaesthesia.

After the session, skin appears slightly reddish and the redness may last from one hour to a day depending on the individual skin's responsiveness and the intensity of the treatment. Afterwards, almost no desquamation is visible and the skin feels already polished to the touch and is visibly brighter.

However, the patient must apply total sun protection cream or gel.

Radiofrequency has been used for many years, especially in skin rejuvenation treatments to induce thermo-stimulation of the dermis. It develops deep heat which determines a shortening of collagen fibres, with a slight lifting effect visible even after the first session, and stimulates the release of cytokines and peptides that favour the formation of new collagen type 1, which has the effect of skin rejuvenation.

Finally, it stimulates dermal microcirculation with greater oxygen and nutrient input, activating the skin cell metabolism.

All this can be useful in improving both the signs of skin aging and acne scarring.

In conclusion, fractional radiofrequency proved to be a safe, gentle but effective treatment for many skin conditions including acne, acne marks and superficial scarring, and leads to rapid skin improvement without the discomfort associated with the evident desquamation caused by chemical peeling.

PHOTODYNAMIC THERAPY

Photodynamic therapy uses a photosensitising substance which reacts to specific wavelengths of light.

The substance, incorporated in a cream, is applied to the skin for a variable time so that it is absorbed. The patient is then exposed to the specific light radiation (blue and/or red light).

This results in chemical reactions with massive release of free radicals and partial skin necrosis. The substance used is aminolevulinic acid (ALA).

The main target in photodynamic therapy for acne is **Propionibacterium acnes**, which already produces a photosensitising molecule called coproporphyrin, making the bactericidal action of the therapy more effective.

The secondary targets are the **sebaceous glands** as the ALA accumulates inside them. They are also partially damaged and sebaceous secretion is reduced, but only temporarily.

During the irradiation, which is a few minutes long, the patient experiences a more or less intense burning sensation. After the session, there is a noticeable reddening of the skin (as it happens after a chemical peeling) with a slight swelling. In the first few days, there might be a worsening of pimples and sebaceous secretion and from the fourth to the tenth day, an evident exfoliation appears. Acne improves afterwards.

Photodynamic therapy for acne is almost ineffective on comedones, but it is particularly effective on papulopustular forms where the presence of PA is greater.

In any case, it is a laborious and long treatment which requires a lot of sessions with a few weeks wait between one and another.

It produces benefits comparable to those of chemical peeling, but having a slight or no effect on the comedones: unlike peeling, there is no deep skin cleansing action.

As in post-peeling, the formation of scabs occurs followed by a visible exfoliation.

A softer treatment uses only blue light (400-500 nanometres wavelength) or both red and blue light which is irradiated on the face for about 20-30 minutes.

Patients do not generally experience burning or discomfort during the session and the following days.

Since it is less aggressive than the actual photodynamic therapy, the treatment should be repeated every week for several weeks in order to obtain visible results and improve pimples: the number of sessions depends on the severity of the acne clinical picture.

However, maintenance cycles or subsequent sessions are required each month.

STEP V: AVOID ALL MISTAKES THAT WORSEN PIMPLES

He that can have patience can have what he will.
Benjamin Franklin (inventor)

Sometimes the treatment for acne does not work; sometimes there are mistakes to avoid when treating pimples. In some cases, minor but important factors are neglected in order to get quick and visible benefits in eliminating pimples.

Sometimes, although you are following the anti-acne therapy recommended by the dermatologist, pimples get worse.

In this case, you interrupt the therapy and blame the dermatologist. Indeed, it might be his/her fault if he/she did not prepare an adequate therapy scheme, if he/she did not give you proper support and advice on treating pimples or if he/she did not tell you what mistakes you need to avoid when treating them.

Sometimes you wanted to do what you want and tried a new product or products.

In all cases, this is like taking one step forward and two steps backwards. In the best scenario, the benefits of the anti-acne therapy will be much slower, but the worst scenario often prevails: acne continues to worsen.

Here are 12 mistakes that make pimple worse:

1) Moisturising creams

Fat and acneic skin does not need to be hydrated, even when it appears dry in some areas (see asphyxiated skin: only the stratum corneum thickens and stratifies) or becomes slightly dry due to the effect of therapies (as with retinoids or exfoliants).

Hydration means swelling the pores cells and causing more obstruction and formation of blackheads and whiteheads.

2) Make-up with coloured creams

When you have acne, you want to mask and make the pimples invisible at all costs. This is perfectly understandable.

Unfortunately, applying foundation and coloured creams (with moisturising effect) makes pimples magically disappear, but it inevitably clogs the pores.

3) Chlorhexidine or antiseptic cleansers

Acne is thought to be an infection but it is not. Indeed, bacteria present on the skin, especially Propionibacterium acnes, cause and aggravate acne inflammation, but it is not necessary to use antiseptic or bactericidal cleansers several times a day. It is one of the mistakes to avoid when treating pimples because it changes the skin's ecosystem: also the "good" bacteria which are normally present on the skin are excessively eliminated and this favours the spread and multiplication of potentially more harmful bacteria or fungi.

4) Sulphur soap

Sulphur has a drying and exfoliating effect so, when you use sulphur soap, your skin looks less dull and shiny and pimples improve. But usually, after ten days, the skin tends to become irritated, pimples appear more inflamed or, in the best case scenario, the skin becomes excessively dry.

In the short term, Sulphur purifies and improves fatty and acneic skin, but in the medium term, it makes skin worse, causing thickening and inflammation.

5) Cleansers and products with glycolic acid and hydroxyacids

Glycolic acid and other acids belonging to the group of hydroxy acids can be incorporated (with low concentrations) in cleansers and anti-acne products for their exfoliating and acidifying action, but unfortunately, they often have an irritating effect on sensitive acneic skin, worsening acne inflammation. Moreover, these molecules also have a hyperhydrating effect and may favour the clogging of the pores, with a worsening of pimples.

6) Neutral soap

A typical mistake is the use of neutral soap: it is thought that since it is 'neutral', it should be gentle and respectful of the skin, but that is not the case. Neutral soap, in contact with water, takes up an alkaline pH and this causes the loss of normal mild acidity of the skin, which guarantees a better protection from bacterial and fungal agents and chemicals: skin balance is lost, pimples form and become more inflamed.

7) Scrubs in case of papulopustular acne

If used gently, granular cleansers or scrubs may be useful in non-inflamed comedonal acne, but they may cause micro-abrasions in papules and pustules, worsening the degree of inflammation and favouring bacterial proliferation.

8) Cortisone creams or lotions

Cortisone-based drugs are powerful anti-inflammatory drugs that, in rare cases, can be used for infiltration into deep scars and pimples (nodulo-cystic acne).

Using cortisone-based creams or lotions can quickly give you a huge benefit in acne, but it is really a big mistake for two reasons:

1. as soon as you suspend the application, you will experience a serious worsening of acne
2. and if you continue or will continue to apply cortisone, you will notice the appearance of new and many blackheads and whiteheads (comedones) that will turn into pimples (steroid acne).

9) Squeezing whiteheads

When you feel and see your skin full of many "small cysts under the skin", the temptation to squeeze them to make them disappear and clean the skin is strong. Unlike blackheads or open comedones, whiteheads or closed comedones are deep.

While removing blackheads with a certain procedure (see later in the text) can be useful, squeezing whiteheads only causes damage:

- whiteheads "burst" under the skin and form deep pimples
- skin is damaged so much that it causes the formation of a persistent spot or even a permanent mark (scar).

In any case, the acne and appearance of your face will worsen, thus obtaining the opposite effect. It is better to be patient and give time to retinoids or exfoliants to perform their action or undergo chemical peeling or exfoliating fractional radiofrequency or sessions for faster results.

10) Sun oils

Everybody knows that in the summer you have to protect your skin from the sun with appropriate products. Sun creams are often fat and make the skin greasy. Oil sprays, instead, since they are liquid, are more spreadable and handy, and seem to make the skin less greasy.

However, they often have comedogenic effects and cause the formation of comedones. Not immediately, but after the summer months, when you return from holidays, you will notice worsening of the skin and an increased number of pimples.

11) Sun lamps

With the sun, but also with sun lamps, acne apparently improves: with the tan, pimples are less visible and it reduces the inflammation to some extent

However, the skin reacts to UV rays by triggering a defence mechanism: the stratum corneum thickens and the occlusion of the pores tends to worsen. Therefore, even in this case, there may be a short-term improvement, which will be though followed by a worsening of pimples.

12) Gel or lotion containing alcohol

Alcohol degreases the skin a lot, possibly too much. In the past, toners or wipes containing alcohol to cleanse were used to clean the skin and remove the grease.

Removing a large part of the hydrolipidic film, the so-called rebound effect occurs: after a few hours, the sebaceous secretion increases and the skin becomes greasier and shinier than before, and then acne also worsens.

Even now there are products that contain traces of alcohol (including gels and antibiotic lotions for acne) that often cause irritation and worsening of pimples inflammation.

As you have noticed, using unsuitable cosmetics is the first sabotaging action on the anti-acne treatments effects.

It is pointless to begin fighting against pimples and follow the best anti-acne cure in the world if you then use unsuitable cosmetics that neutralise the action of the recommended treatments. That is why it is mandatory to set up proper cosmetic habits, starting from make-up.

5 RULES TO MASK PIMPLES WITHOUT DAMAGE

Masking or covering pimples is a much felt need for acne sufferers. Often, when new pimples appear on the face, the first concern is that their duration is as short as possible.

In fact, even the best pimples remedies cannot make them disappear over hours but only over days – and they are not always so effective.

For this reason, the acne sufferer can feel they need to cover pimples with various make-up products.

Masking pimples is like knocking down acne from one day to another: although it is hard, making pimples invisible has many benefits from a psychological point of view.

Some dermatological studies confirm that this alleviates the psychological suffering of patients, "magically" boosts mood and self-esteem, and reduces the degree of acne inflammation. **It ultimately determines an improvement of acne**, even without any dermatological care.

However, it all depends on the cosmetic products you use, because you may also be able to quickly mask pimples very well but then obtain a major acne deterioration in the next few days or weeks.

In order to properly cover pimples, you should first use a green or beige stick concealer on the individual pimples, then a foundation on the whole face to match the colour of your skin, and then (but not necessarily) a covering compact powder.

In this way, you would obtain a perfect camouflage, but you would inevitably occlude the pores of your skin!

So, what are the rules to follow?

Here are the 5 rules to cover pimples:

1. **Do not ever use products which cover too much**: when you can, avoid stick concealers. Although they are effective, they contain waxes that close the pores.

2. **Do not use coloured creams** with a moisturising effect as a foundation: your oily skin does not need to be moisturised. As I explained before, the pores cells would swell and this would contribute to the occlusion of the pores.

3. **Do not use oil-free lotions or similar** as a foundation: they should be the ideal product for oily and acneic skin but, in fact, they are not really oil free, they are emulsions (with a high percentage of powder) where the liquid part is made up of water and fatty substances that can still have a moisturising effect. Sometimes they can also contain small amounts of alcohol, which would lead to an irritating action.

What can you do to cover pimples without worsening acne?

4. **Use only covering compact powders**: these are compact creams made up in a small part by a cream or emulsion and in a greater part by a fine coloured powder that remains on the surface without occluding the pores. The percentage of creamy emulsion is so small that it ensures the product's spreadability, but without having a considerable moisturising effect.

5. **Choose "oil free" compact powders** where the oil percentage is really reduced to the minimum necessary, at the expense of spreadability and covering effectiveness. In any case, they would be the ideal product for camouflage and make-up for acneic skin, when pimples are not very large and inflamed.

HOW TO SHAVE WITHOUT IRRITATING PIMPLES

In young men with acne, shaving with a standard or electric razor could cause a worsening of pimples.

Some people with very sensitive skin cannot tolerate the use of electric razor, while others find the standard razor more irritating.

In both cases, shaving always represents a slight trauma for acneic skin for 5 reasons:

1. Due to the presence of pimples, the skin surface is not smooth but irregular and this causes a high chance of cuts or micro-abrasions
2. Inflammation is amplified by shaving micro-traumas
3. Micro-cuts may favour the implantation of other bacteria that cause further inflammation

4. Foam or shaving cream may contain surfactants and irritating substances, as well as emolliating/moisturising.
5. After-shave products may contain alcohol (and we have seen the imbalance that this substance can cause on hydrolipidic film and sebaceous secretion) and/or moisturising substances that may be comedogenic.

It is therefore appropriate to follow some rules in order to reduce these factors as much as possible:

- limit the frequency of shaving: do it on alternate days
- shave gently in order to avoid micro-traumas
- use an electric razor with flexible head that continuously fits to the contours of your face, without exerting excessive pressure
- if you use a standard razor, use a foam or shaving gel containing antiseptic and emollient substances.
- choose an electric razor with flexible head so that it fits the irregularities of the skin surface and avoid shaving "against the growth".
- when you are done with/after shaving, wash your face with the cleanser recommended by your dermatologist in order to remove any shaving product residue, reduce bacterial charge and rebalance the skin.
- using an after-shave product should be superfluous when you have oily skin, and might be counterproductive in acne skin: in fact you would not need to hydrate, and washing your face with the proper detergent has already a soothing and rebalance effect.
- in the presence of inflamed acne lesions, it is appropriate and necessary to apply an antibiotic/antiseptic gel after shaving.

HOW TO REMOVE BLACK HEADS CORRECTLY

Removing blackheads is a very common temptation.
It is very easy to squeeze blackheads and then "free the pores", but it is less easy to avoid causing:

- the inflammation of the pilosebaceous follicle accelerating the appearance of the pimple
- an infection caused by the bacteria already present on your

skin or carried by your hands
- the formation of spots, or even bumps of the skin that look like very dilated pores but they are small scars instead.

Squeezing pimples, as well as squeezing blackheads, can also cause permanent damage to your face skin.

If we need to do it, it is important to do it correctly and without causing complications.
- first, wash your face with a cleanser specific for acne with acidic pH, preferably if containing rebalancing-soothing and bacteriostatic substances, and rinse with warm (but not too much) water to dilate the pores.
- disinfect your hands and the affected area with alcohol
- take a cotton bud dampened with alcohol and exert pressure on the skin at the sides of the comedo in order to gently squeeze the sebum content and cellular debris.

Why not squeeze blackheads with your fingers? Because nails, even when short and clean, may carry germs and cause a greater trauma. The cotton bud is smaller than your fingers, more effective and precise in exerting pressure.

- do not insist on squeezing the blackhead until blood comes out; stop before causing dermis small capillaries collapse or follicle breaking that can lead to inflammation and deep pimples in the treated area.
- wipe the surface of the skin and disinfect with a cotton bud dampened with alcohol.
- apply an antibiotic gel or lotion immediately after, repeat 2 times over the next 24 hours.

In order to eliminate blackheads and avoid the sudden appearance of pimples and holes on the skin, it is important not to skip any of these steps.

STEP VI: THE ANTI-ACNE DIET

You have made the first steps, you have done the exercises, you have decided to win against acne, you have started to act with determination, you have improved your motivation by giving yourself goals every day.

You have finally started dermatological treatments.

However, as we have seen, it is not enough to act only "superficially". If we want to achieve long-lasting and stable results, we must begin to act right away also from the inside, on our metabolic processes, and this necessarily requires longer times.

We are at step VI.

Now is the time to take care of your diet.

As we have seen, the influence of diet on acne has always been controversial: do some foods actually cause acne worsening or breakouts?

There are those who think there is no link and that is just a coincidence or a popular belief, and there are those who have always given credit to this ancient intuition that, as in many other cases, has some truth.

However, many scientific studies have not yet confirmed these beliefs.

Something has recently changed: at least, today some studies tell us that nutrition has nothing to do with acne and some others say that *a certain type of diet and certain foods* can *negatively (or positively) affect the acneic inflammatory process.*

It is important to point out that these studies do not state that the diet causes acne, but that a given type of diet may aggravate its inflammatory state. They are also related to other studies where a certain type of diet is said to increase the inflammatory state of your body. (I recommend you to go back and read the chapter on nutrition as a secondary factor.)

After all, the skin is the largest organ of our body, why should we not eat foods to take care of our skin?

Our body is a sophisticated chemical laboratory in which chemical substances introduced with food are constantly transformed and reworked. These substances are used to build our cells, our blood and all organs and apparatus: we are (and we become) what we eat.

If you think about it, even drugs are substances that we introduce from the outside and that interact with the chemistry of our organism by modifying it (for better or worse).

With nutrition, we can change and improve the quality of our tissues and organs. If we are what we eat, even the state of our skin will reflect the quality of our diet.

At this stage, we therefore begin to learn and avoid food containing low quality and harmful molecules because they are pro-inflammatory (they stimulate the formation of toxic substances that raise the degree of our body's inflammation).

Indeed, it will take some time for these chemicals to be eliminated and replaced by better and healthier molecules (mostly with an anti-inflammatory effect).

The purpose is to reduce acne inflammation over time in order to avoid prolonged and repeated antibiotic therapies, with all the side effects they may have and which would nevertheless yield only transient results.

Just because the benefits will be visible in the medium-long term, it is advisable to start as soon as possible.

Now the **basic skills (and knowledge)** to develop or improve are:

- how to activate the normal purifying functions of the body
- how to choose the right foods

in order to achieve **intermediate goals**, you should:

- avoid proinflammatory feeding
- improve the skin through an anti-inflammatory diet

I will outline the general concepts of an adequate anti-acne nutrition with some practical tips, but I would like to point out that:

a. although the information can be useful, they do not substitute in any way your doctor and other specialists' advice and prescriptions or a nutritionist's guidance;
b. before making any changes to your diet, it is always necessary to consider the assessments of your health status and the

opinions of your doctor and other specialists who are taking care of you;

c. "DIY" diets can do more harm than good.

Therefore, I strongly advise you to consult a nutritionist who is experienced in detoxifying and anti-acne diets.

If you are overweight, this is absolutely essential.

In any case, it is important to keep your body weight under control in order to prevent hormonal imbalances linked to the increase in adipose tissue and involved in the pathogenesis of acne.

WHY AND HOW SOME FOODS MAKE PIMPLES WORSE

We eat a lot of chocolate or sweets, we drink beer, wine or other alcoholic drinks and the following day the number and size of the pimples increase visibly.

From personal experience, every person affected by acne knows that some foods cause a sudden worsening of this disease.

Here, I will summarise and deepen concepts already outlined in the chapter on nutrition as a secondary factor, but focusing on specific foods that can alleviate it and those that can, instead, exacerbate the acne inflammation.

The "bad" foods can act through 2 mechanisms:
1. **they increase blood sugar (and insulin) too quickly**
2. **they contain or cause the release of histamine**

The end result is always an increase in the general inflammation of the body.

Let us analyse the first factor.

In 2007, a study published on American Journal of Clinical Nutrition came to the conclusion that a diet based on high glycemic index foods (i.e. foods rich in refined sugars) is correlated to a greater severity of acne lesions.

The **glycemic index** (GI) is the ability of a food to increase blood sugar levels more or less rapidly.

Let us remember what happens when blood sugar suddenly increases.

As a result, there is a more or less intense stimulus to insulin secretion from the pancreas, and insulin is the hormone that stores sugars in fat reserves, making people gain weight.

Foods based on high glycemic index foods determine a continuous excess of insulin in the blood.

As we have seen, this also causes greater presence of male hormones and an increased production of arachidonic acid and "bad" inflammatory eicosanoids. This triggers a chain of events that lead to the chronic picture of silent inflammation, accompanied by further hormonal imbalances (increase in cortisol and male hormones).

In this case, if we measure blood sugar, it may also result "normal" due to insulin secretion – but insulin levels have increased, instead.

Once again, all this can explain the worsening of acne.

In the same research mentioned earlier, a remarkable reduction in pimples and inflammation of acne was observed after 3 months of a diet richer in proteins and low glycemic index foods.

The result was comparable to that achieved with the continuous use of gel and antibiotic creams.

If you want to improve the quality of your nutrition, you should go back and reflect on the concept of glycemic index.

The glycemic index (GI) is a system which assesses the quality of carbohydrates, based on a score of 0 to 100, where the highest values are attributed to foods that cause the fastest increase in blood sugar.

The reference point is pure sugar, which has a glycemic index of 100.

It indicates the rate of entry of sugars into the blood stream, which may also be influenced by the mode of consumption or the way the food has been cooked.

To be precise, the glycemic index is important but, for practical purposes, the concept of glycemic load of a food is even more useful.

The **glycemic load** (GL) takes into account the quality of the carbohydrate (hence the GI) and the amount in grams present in the average portion of a given food.

It is calculated by multiplying the grams of carbohydrates present in an average portion by the GI.

The glycemic load then tells us that we should not only consider the quality of the carbohydrates we ingest, but we should also be careful about the quantity.

The fundamental concept is this: it is far better to have **a mild, slow and gradual rise in blood sugar and an equally slow and gradual decrease** than frequent and sudden short-lived increases. Glycemic peaks lead to insulin peaks that drastically lower blood sugar and do not create any lasting sense of satiety.

After a few dozen minutes, we are hungry again and this urgently pushes us to eat other high glycemic index foods in order to "feel better and boost energy levels". In this way, a real psychophysical addiction to such foods and a dangerous vicious circle are created.

The end result is that insulin levels constantly remain high, with the toxic consequences described above.

Even milk and derivatives contain substances that stimulate the release of insulin.

In the May 2008 issue of the Journal of the American Academy of Dermatology, an article highlighted that teens who were drinking too much milk were affected by more severe forms of acne.

High levels of progesterone and IGF-1 (insulin-like-growth-factor) may be present in milk, which has an insulin-like action in favouring an increased availability of male hormones and causing a worsening of the inflammatory state.

Also for this reason, as we will see soon, milk chocolate (unlike dark chocolate) worsens the pimples.

It is therefore a fact that some foods can cause a worsening of the pimples, varying from individual to individual.

For example, let us take one of the most "incriminated" foods: chocolate. The belief that chocolate causes the appearance of pimples is a very common myth and has always been a very discussed issue in the dermatological field.

In an Italian study, published a few years ago on the Journal of the American Academy of Dermatology, scientists attempted to determine whether chocolate causes the appearance of pimples. A group of 205 patients aged between 10 and 24 was examined and it was confirmed that there is no link between chocolate consumption and acne: there is no influence on the production and composition of sebaceous secretion and chocolate does not affect the evolution of this skin disease.

Let us stop for a moment and see the positive or negative effects that chocolate has on our skin and body.

In fact, distinctions should be made.

Dark chocolate (at least 70% pure) is really beneficial because is rich in antioxidants: compared to milk chocolate, the amount of polyphenols is much higher.

We can recognise the presence of polyphenols from the bitter and astringent taste, regardless the declared percentage of cocoa in the tablet.

Cocoa polyphenols are distinguished in 3 groups: Catechins (about 37%), Anthocyanins (4%) and Proanthocyanidins (58%).

We know that a high polyphenols intake helps decreasing the onset of cardiovascular diseases such as heart attack and stroke.

Polyphenols act by:
- reducing platelets coagulation
- inhibiting lipoproteins oxidation
- free radical scavenger action ("sweeping away free radicals")
- modulating "bad" or pro-inflammatory eicosanoids (prostaglandins, thromboxanes and leukotrienes) in order to inhibit the reaction of arachidonic acid transformation.

People who eat small amounts of dark chocolate daily have a relatively lower level of C-Reactive Protein (CRP= unspecified inflammation index) than others.

Dark chocolate polyphenols thus reduce the overall inflammatory state.

But be careful: **it all depends on the type and quantity of the chocolate you eat!**

Chocolate causes pimples, or make them worse, if it is milk or white chocolate or eaten daily in given quantities.

In fact, milk and white chocolate contain a large amount of fat and sugar that can raise blood sugar and worsen the silent chronic inflammatory state.

According to clinical studies, only a small dose of dark chocolate (6-7 g a day) may be useful as a general anti-inflammatory and does not cause or worsen pimples.

Excessive daily amounts of chocolate determine an excessive glycemic load and a **release of histamine** and other pro-inflammatory chemical mediators that, in particularly sensitive patients, cause a worsening of the overall inflammatory state.

If your skin is already inflamed by acne, chocolate may still lead to a further worsening of pimples.

Chocolate can thus amplify the overall and skin inflammatory state through both of the two mechanisms mentioned above.

Let us now look at the second mechanism through which some foods may make acne inflammation worse: let us see what other foods are rich in histamine or histamine-liberators.

Histamine is a chemical agent widely spread in our body and plays a leading role in inflammatory and allergic responses (e.g. urticaria). A massive release of histamine in the body can also cause very serious and dangerous reactions such as anaphylactic shock.

Histamine stimulates vasodilation (redness), itching and swelling, increasing the passage of fluids and inflammatory cells through the blood vessels and into tissues.

And **if acne inflammation is already present, histamine will amplify it.**

FOODS RICH IN HISTAMINE OR HISTAMINE-LIBERATORS

- Strawberries, citrus fruits, bananas, pineapple, raspberries, avocado
- Peanuts, nuts, hazelnuts and almonds
- Beans, lentils, beans, peas, chickpeas
- Tomatoes, spinach, potato starch
- Fermented cheese, yoghurt, brewer's yeast
- Egg white, chocolate
- Pork and sausages, canned foods, stock cubes
- Fermented drinks (wine, beer), cola, coffee
- Spices, food preservatives such as benzoates (benzoic acid and its salts)
- Crustaceans, preserved fish (herring, algae, sardines, salmon, tuna)

When ingested, these foods and additives release histamine, or release it along with other inflammation chemical mediators, causing degranulation of mast cells and basophil granulocytes (inflammatory cells in the dermis and other tissues).

In the above list, as you can see, there are several foods that have always been "blacklisted" as they trigger acne.

However, each of us is different and responds differently to these small amounts of histamine.

There is a varying degree of sensitivity; some people are particularly susceptible and can even be histamine intolerant, others can be little or non-responsive.

Inflammatory or pseudo-allergic events in response to certain foods may therefore vary from mild to severe ailments. The diamine oxidase enzyme (DAO) is involved in the degradation of histamine in the intestinal tract and therefore helps to eliminate it before it enters the circulatory system.

Some individuals produce few diamine oxidase, some others do not.

Certainly, it is known that alcohol inhibits DAOs thus enhancing inflammatory disorders related to the histamine release in predisposed subjects.

Have you noticed the appearance of new pimples or their worsening following the ingestion of wine, beer, and spirits?

In fact, alcohol stimulates the overall and skin inflammation.

Can you see how everything can be connected?

However, there is good news: you can act against acne also from the inside, not only with drugs, but also with the "most natural" existing drug that you use every day: food.

HOW TO DETOX

written in collaboration with Dr Sara Barletta, biologist nutritionist and responsible for the Nutrition section of our blog.

We strongly advise you to follow an anti-acne diet as a natural remedy to help control acne in the long term.

Summing up, we have seen how we should absolutely avoid or reduce the consumption of foods that:

1. raise blood sugar (and insulin) levels too quickly
2. contain or cause release of histamine

The maintenance of normal insulin levels can be achieved by rebalancing our diet and consuming:

- in larger amounts, low glycemic index foods
- in moderate amounts, average glycemic index foods
- and avoiding high glycemic index foods or reducing their amount to minimum.

If we are not willing to settle for junk living,
we certainly should not settle for junk food.
Sally Edwards (athlete)

Luckily, there is no junk food in the traditional Mediterranean diet and it also includes many of the low glycemic index foods.

We already mentioned the concepts of glycemic index and glycemic load.

There is no simple way of predicting foods' glycemic index because it does not only depend on the mode of consumption, but also on the way they are cooked and combined together. For instance, fats and proteins reduce the glycemic index of many carbohydrate-rich foods such as pasta.

If you want to find out the glycemic index of a particular food, you can consult the Univeristy of Sidney website www.glycemicindex.com

For a precise and personalised anti-acne diet plan, it is always good to consult an experienced nutritionist of this field. In this section, though, we will give you some indications and basic examples on glycemic index, foods to be avoided or introduced in your diet, and a 3 day detox diet plan, which you can either follow or use as a reference point, if you have no particular disorder or illness.

If you are in doubt, we strongly advise you to contact your doctor or nutritionist.

So let us start making some adjustments to your eating habits through a real detox phase, with the aim of cleans your body from toxins like free radicals and pro-inflammatory eicosanoids, histamine, and caffeine-based drinks that worsen emotional stress.

FOODS TO AVOID OR REDUCE TO MINIMUM

- sugar
- other high glycemic index foods (GI > 70): e.g. jam, pasta, white bread, white rice, refined white flour, carrots, potatoes, polenta, gnocchi, honey, cornflakes, dried biscuits, kiwi, banana, crackers, biscuits, sweets, ice creams, sugary beverages
- junk food: pancakes, fries and buns, other foods fried or rich in refined sugars and saturated fats (butter, lard)
- alcoholic beverages: you can have a glass of wine or a beer every now and then, if you are not particularly sensitive to histamine.
- milk chocolate and cocoa creams
- fermented milk and cheese (gorgonzola, camembert, etc.)

FOODS TO CONSUME WITH MODERATION

- medium glycemic index foods (GI between 55 and 70): e.g. wholemeal flour, egg pasta, oranges, dried bacon beans
- foods rich in histamine or that stimulate histamine release. We inserted them in this list because you might be a little or non-sensitive to histamine and some of these foods also contain omega 3 and other beneficial substances for acne (so, do not be surprised that you will also find them among the highly recommended foods). Other foods, instead, are also found among those you should avoid.

On a case by case basis, you will need to evaluate your skin reaction to these foods. So, we show you the list again, because it is necessary to see if some of these foods make your acne worse or cause other ailments (e.g. itching or mild nausea).

- Strawberries, citrus fruits, bananas, pineapple, raspberries, avocado
- Peanuts, nuts, hazelnuts and almonds
- Beans, lentils, beans, peas, chickpeas
- Tomatoes, spinach, potato starch
- Fermented cheese, yoghurt, brewer's yeast
- Egg white, chocolate
- Pork and sausages, canned foods, stock cubes

- Fermented drinks (wine, beer), cola, coffee
- Spices, food preservatives such as benzoates (benzoic acid and its salts)
- Crustaceans, preserved fish (herring, algae, sardines, salmon, tuna)

We therefore recommend you to keep a **food diary** for at least two weeks, where you can write down your meals and snacks and any possible worsening, and share it with your dermatologist and nutritionist.

If you notice that a specific food causes an increase in inflammation and pimples, please remove it from the diet for at least 4 weeks, and check if your skin improves.

If you daily reduce or avoid high glycemic index and histamine-rich foods (if you are sensitive to them), your body and skin would experience a real detoxifying revolution. But we can do a lot more by following a healthier and more energising diet.

You will soon see which foods you can introduce in your diet or consume more in order to reduce the overall inflammation, improve pimples and prevent acne.

But first, let us go back to the role of omega 3 in acne and why foods rich in omega 3 are highly recommended in an anti-acne diets.

We have already talked about omega 3: they are essential fatty acids – our body does not produce them and we can only introduce them with food. They make the cellular membrane phospholipids less rigid, thus promoting metabolic exchanges and keeping them young. But the most important action of omega 3 is precisely in the antioxidant action and in promoting the production of "good" eicosanoids i.e. anti-inflammatory.

Human beings have evolved following a diet based on a ratio of omega 6 to omega 3 of about 1:1. Many scientists believe that brain development and intelligence in humans have been accelerated by the high consumption of fish and foods rich in omega 3.

Nutritionists estimate that the modern Western diet is completely unbalanced in favour of omega 6 with a ratio of 15:1.

This means there is a serious omega 3 deficiency and an excess of omega 6.

Let us briefly remember that Omega 6 generates **arachidonic acid** and, from this, **gamma linoleic acid (GLA)** and **dihomo-gamma-linolenic acid (DGLA)**, which are precursors of both "good" eicosanoids with anti-inflammatory action and "bad" eicosanoids with pro-inflammatory action. While omega 3, **eicosapentaenoic acid (EPA)** and **docosahexaenoic acid (DHA)** only produce "good" eicosanoids, with a powerful anti-inflammatory effect.

Why is it important to take the right amount of essential fatty acids with foods and balance the ratio between omega 3 and omega 6?

When our diet is too rich in omega 6 (compared to omega 3), cellular metabolic reactions are mostly directed towards their massive transformation into arachidonic acid: for this reason, pro-inflammatory eicosanoids and silent chronic inflammation prevail in our body.

If you are taking omega 3-rich foods or supplements you will correct the food and metabolic imbalance, thus increasing the production of anti-inflammatory eicosanoids.

The addition of omega 3 to the diet will gradually improve the quality of the sebum produced, less subject to oxidation, less susceptible to atmospheric oxygen, and then less pro-inflammatory: comedogenesis and acne inflammation will tend to reduce.

RECOMMENDED FOODS

- **low glycemic index foods** (GI < 55): e.g. pearl barley, spaghetti*, dried lentils, dried chickpeas, apple, pear, peach and cherry
- **lean meat**, preferably **white**
- **cured meat** like ham or speck

Did you know that their particular shape reduces the speed of sugars absorption, even better if they are cooked 'al dente'?

- **Water**: Drink plenty of water (preferably not sparkling), at least 2 litres per day. They correspond to about 10 to 12 glasses. Water helps to purify the body and also to improve the hydration and metabolism of the skin. You can also help with herbal teas and consuming water-rich foods such as watermelon, melon and cucumber.

- **Foods rich in omega-3 fatty acids:**
  - Salmon, mackerel, fresh anchovies and sardines
  - Flax seeds and flaxseed oil
  - Chia seeds
  - Nuts, almonds
  - Hemp oil
  - Algae

- **Foods rich in antioxidants (many fruits and vegetables):**
  - Melons, oranges, tomatoes, cherries and strawberries (rich in vitamin C)
  - Vegetable oils, hazelnuts, soya, almonds, green leafy vegetables (rich in vitamin E)
  - Broccoli and spinach (vitamin A, B, C, K, E)
  - Infused green tea 2 or 3 times a day (rich in polyphenols)
  - Artichokes (vitamin C) with purifying effect on the liver
  - Extra virgin olive oil (rich in vitamin E) for seasoning salads and vegetables
  - Seasonal fruit and vegetable smoothies (see recipes later)

- **Vitamin A-rich foods:**

-      Apricots, mangoes, carrots, tomatoes, pumpkin, bell peppers, melons, kiwis, eggs, dandelion, chilli pepper, cod liver oil, rocket or other dark leafy vegetables.

These foods are rich in beta-carotene, a precursor of vitamin A or retinol, whose derivatives (retinoids) represent the most powerful anti-acne drugs: they counteract comedogenesis.

- **Probiotic foods**
-      Probiotic yoghurt without added sugars (bacterial species Lactobacillus rhamnosus, acidophilus and Bifidobacterium) have an anti-inflammatory and normalizing action on sebum and skin pH.

Smoothies and detoxifying and purifying infusions

Apples, carrot and ginger smoothie
Ingredients: 100 g apple, 100 g carrot, 10 g ginger, water (to taste). Method: wash and coarse chop and apple, carrot and ginger. Blend the ingredients. Dilute with water.
Option 2: Replace the apple with 100 g of seasonal fruit. You should drink the smoothie immediately in order to reduce the vitamins oxidation contained in the fruits.

Artichoke, melissa and lime infuse
Ingredients: still water, 1 fresh artichoke, 1 organic lime, melissa.
Method: Boil 500 ml of water with fresh artichoke leaves for about 10 minutes. Turn off the flame, add melissa, grated lime peel and leave to infuse for another 10 minutes. Filter the infusion, add lime juice and drink it warm.

EXAMPLE OF 3 DAY DETOX PLAN:

Day 1
Breakfast: Probiotic yoghurt + 200 g of fresh pineapple smoothie
Snack: 30 g chia seeds
Lunch: whole pasta with artichokes, cherry tomatoes and basil (recipe*)
Snack: 150 g of red berries

Dinner: salmon with herbs and whole wheat bread coating (recipe*)

Day 2
Breakfast: glass of hot water and lemon + probiotic yoghurt with 20 g of oat bran
Snack: celery, carrot, apple and ginger smoothie
Lunch: quinoa or brown rice with curry, stir-fry vegetables and soy sauce
Snack: 2 cucumbers
Dinner: turkey and speck roll with yoghurt sauce and grilled vegetables
Day 3
Breakfast: low-fat yoghurt with 30 g of muesli
Snack: pink grapefruit juice
Lunch: barley with broccoli and pine nuts cream
Snack: 20 g of almonds
Dinner: chickpeas and potatoes burger with steamed carrots

Please make an effort now, these rules are the starting point: taking small and gradual steps, you will need to start changing your eating habits, adjusting or eliminating some foods and introducing new ones.

Within a few weeks, you should already see improvements not only on acne but also on your body shape. And, if you do not have any particular problems, you will be able to notice an improvement of your skin condition.

In some cases, instead, just because the cleansing mechanisms of your body are set in motion, an initial temporary worsening can occur, but then followed by a more stable improvement.

Do not worry, it is important to proceed along the outlined path with patience and determination.

STEP VII: WIN ACNE WITH "STYLE"

Opportunities multiply as they are seized.
Sun Tzu (military strategist)

The seventh step of this path is not the last.

As I explained to you, you must see it as a circular path in which step VII embraces and reinforces the previous steps.

You cannot cure a chronic disease like acne if you do not have a strong motivation and you do not know how to achieve the goal. You would soon abandon the therapies if you did not have self-esteem and if you would not be able handle the stress of any worsening or setbacks. Choose the right dermatologist and follow the therapies and the prescribed treatments with his/her help.

If you did not know the mistakes to avoid during the treatment, these would be ineffective and if you did not improve your diet, you would not be able to finally put acne inflammation under control over the long term.

You need a method, i.e. what I have described in this book, because your ultimate goal should not be limited to not making the pimples worse or less inflamed, but it is more ambitious: keep your skin free from pimples by learning to treat acne in a global way.

In fact, we can win against acne thanks to a healthier life!

Do you remember that I mentioned the new science of epigenetics earlier? It is not just what we eat that can change the expression of our genes and, consequently, help to cope with chronic inflammation.

As you will learn, recent studies demonstrate the role of exercise and sleep as important regulators of our DNA.

Now the basic skills to develop or improve are:

- how to organise effectively
- how to develop new and healthier habits

in order to achieve intermediate goals:

- build a daily anti-acne routine

- improve your lifestyle

LIFESTYLE

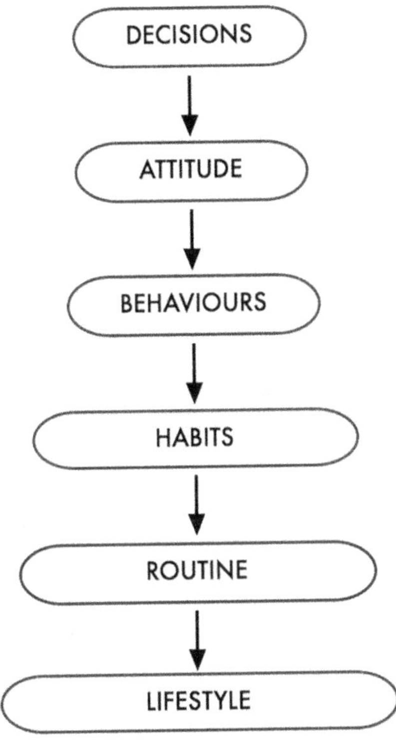

The ultimate goal of the 7 steps path to win against acne is to build what I call an *"anti-acne lifestyle"* in order for you to cure your skin constantly and effortlessly, and making it finally free from pimples.

BUILDING A DAILY ANTI-ACNE ROUTINE

For the things we have to learn before we can do them, we learn by doing them.
Aristotle

Now that you have understood the strategy to follow, it is time to put in practice everything you have learned all together, with a global approach.

Winning against acne requires commitment; in the end, the most effective anti-acne therapies are also the simplest, but the initial phase is always hard.

Like any other new beginning.

In the first step, you saw that:
- real goals have deadlines and are linked to action
- time management, or better, managing your daily tasks is important

In order to organise yourself better, as your goal approaches, we must set a deadline and act.

You would surely like to remove pimples from your face within a few days or weeks, but you must be concrete and patient: it is a result that you can achieve progressively.

Set a realistic and close deadline: seeing your acne improve within 4 weeks.

I think this goal you have agreed with your dermatologist, with whom you have set deadlines for treatments and scheduled a check-up examination (perhaps just 1 month later) should be used to evaluate the effectiveness of the therapies.

Now, the daily management of the treatments is up to you!

However, if you want to see benefits quickly, you need some commitment and discipline: curing your skin must become a habit.

In the end, if you think about it, in order to cure acne, you need to perform actions that require just **a dozen minutes a day** in total.

The problem is that people often tend to underestimate and postpone these small tasks – they are not constant.

How to maintain your anti-acne care commitments by building your own daily anti-acne routine

Dermatological care for pimples or other skin diseases is generally a long process, consisting of various moments and phases, and based on the application of cosmetics, the administration of drugs and food supplements, and possible various outpatient treatments.

Your dermatologist must have prescribed you the treatments with their relevant timing of administration, methods and doses of the products (cosmetics or drugs) to be applied on the skin or taken orally, so you should already have a plan.

The plan is generally divided into several moments of the day: morning, afternoon, evening.

The pillars of a dermatological anti-acne therapy are:

The cleanser

Using a specific cleanser, recommended by the dermatologist and based on your type of acne and skin, you will remove the excess of hydrolipidic film and debris from the stratum corneum, with a soothing, anti-inflammatory and re-balancing effect on your skin's pH.

The evening product

It is usually an exfoliant or antibiotic/antiseptic. Needless to say, the product and the specific active ingredient have been prescribed by the dermatologist according to the type of skin and pimples so I am only describing product categories.

You just need to find time to apply them, always after cleansing – on a cleaner and more receptive skin: the product will be more effective by acting all night long, when the skin is away from the sun and atmospheric agents and is under repair and regeneration.

The morning product

It is generally an antibiotic/antiseptic, always applied after having washed your face.

The phases of a daily routine may seem obvious as the specialist has already written all the instructions...

But that is not so easy. In fact, you will be the only person choosing when to use (or not use) the product – the exact time of the morning, afternoon or evening.

How?

By combining treatments to other everyday tasks so that you can follow them regularly.

This too may seem obvious, but:

how many times did you "skip" the application of the cream?
how many times did you go to sleep without washing your face or removing make-up?
did you forget to take the antibiotic or the food supplement?
Maybe you did not have time or the energy to do so at that time...

One of the key ingredients of therapeutic efficacy is your perseverance.

How do I find time to perform these daily tasks?

Start **organising your regular day** to introduce your "anti-acne" commitments.

1. Get a blank sheet and create a day schedule dividing it into three parts: morning, afternoon and evening
2. Write down your minimum commitments during the various phases of the day
3. Assess your commitments according to importance and urgency criteria in order to establish the priorities: are they important? Are they urgent?
4. You will definitely have to give high priority to anti-acne care
5. Eliminate or reduce some tasks/commitments which are less important than eliminating pimples: make sure you will find time
6. Now, for each phase, identify important and constant (routine) activities and introduce the anti-acne task immediately before or after one of them so that it will be more difficult for you to postpone it. (e.g. a meal, preparing your school bag, studying, brushing your teeth, etc.)

The three questions you should ask yourself for not postponing your anti-acne treatments when important or urgent commitments suddenly come out:

- Is it a commitment that I can postpone?
- Is it an excuse to postpone my anti-acne treatments?
- Is it really something more important than my anti-acne care?

Now take the dermatologist's prescription and go back to the daily plan you have prepared.

In the three phases of the day, introduce:

A. the recommended cosmetics, drugs and food supplements according to your specialist's instructions
B. the meals and snacks recommended by your nutritionist
C. the exercises I have advised in this book.

You will then have a complete outline of your entire anti-acne strategy!

These are key appointments you cannot miss, if you want to see results in your fight against pimples.

Checking the effectiveness of anti-acne treatments day by day

It is important to understand and evaluate the first (both positive and negative) effects of individual products and the overall anti-acne care.

Look at your skin every day to see how it reacts and if, above all, problems arise.

- Does your skin tend to dry out? Little or too much?
- Does it tend to get irritated and red?
- Does it itch?
- Does it burn?
- Is it more sensitive to sun, heat, and cold?

If you experience some excessive skin reaction or worsening of the pimples, you may need to suspend the "suspected" product: perhaps the quantity was too much and you should call your dermatologist to tell him about it and ask for his/her advice.

Evaluate if there are benefits, but do it objectively, without getting obsessed with the ups and downs that you can normally experience. Remember, the single day and the single pimples are not important.

You have to pay attention to the evolution of the overall skin state in terms of weeks.

- Is the skin becoming cleaner?
- Is the number of comedones decreasing?
- Do pimples tend to bleed?

Or

- Are you noticing any improvement?
- Has the number of pimples increased?
- Have deeper pimples appeared?

Please take note, during the next examination, your dermatologist will ask for your impressions on individual products and overall anti-acne care.

This is important information that will help refine the treatment and improve the anti-acne cure.

All these considerations and suggestions may seem obvious to you but trivial and unlikely mistakes in treating acne often make the therapy and the entire path very ineffective.

That is right, anti-acne care is a continuous path: which is why a daily routine is needed.

THE ANTI-ACNE LIFESTYLE

We are what we repeatedly do.
Aristotle

So far, we have seen all you can do to fight against pimples and also things you should not do.

Now, in fact, at the conclusion of our journey, I want to talk about how to go beyond anti-acne care and how to further improve the quality of your life.

I perfectly understand how young people can be full of energy and desire to live. They can have the inclination to rebel against rules and discipline.

When health and wellbeing are involved, though, we should understand that there are principles that are valid for everyone, which have to do with the optimal functioning of our body.

You are always free to follow or ignore them.

The main secret of a healthy and happy life, and therefore better life, is this one: **have respect for yourself.**

In regards to your anti-acne path, this means that you should not harm yourself, your body, and your skin with harmful habits but rather respect them by looking after yourself regularly.

If you stress your body with drugs and stimulants, lead a very irregular life (from nutrition to sleep), have negative thoughts and attitudes, or spend your days at home in front of the TV, how do you think your skin will look? Will your acne be more severe or less severe?

If you have read this book carefully, you know the answer. In fact, we have already seen how some factors concerning lifestyle, smoking, diet, and stress can heavily affect the skin's beauty and health.

So, now it is time to consider 4 factors that lay the foundations of a healthier and more balanced life:

- Regular sleep
- Regular exercise
- A healthy fun lifestyle
- A healthy attitude

As you have already guessed, they all have an indirect but significant impact on acne.

GOOD SLEEP

When we sleep, our brain, like a computer, resets itself and tidies up its memory, "files" and connections.

This happens at all ages, but during adolescence this process of regeneration and remodelling is even more important and deeper. It is the basis of mental clarity, the ability to solve problems, and creativity. If this process were consistently insufficient or disturbed (as in the total deprivation of sleep used in some forms of torture), our computer would start running badly until it goes haywire.

We all know that poor quality or quantity of sleep can reduce the efficiency of our brain. This also creates a condition of psychological stress that, when prolonged, raises cortisol levels in the blood causing acne or making it worse.

Stress greatly affects the quality of sleep: a dangerous vicious circle is thus created.

So, what to do to enjoy a restful and regenerating sleep?

In the late afternoon, avoid carrying out activities that over-stimulate your mind:

- drink coffee and alcohol
- smoking
- watching TV
- intense physical activity

Avoid altering sleep-wake rhythm:

- sleeping too much in the afternoon (but a short siesta of up to 30 minutes can be regenerating)
- going to sleep very late in the evening and prolonging sleep until late morning: in this way, you completely mess up your biological clock
- sleeping more than 8 hours

REGULAR PHYSICAL ACTIVITY

In addition to the long-term health benefits, exercise also benefits the skin because it favours blood flow, with increased oxygen and nutrients, and the elimination of cellular metabolic waste products: skin becomes brighter and fresher.

Physical activity is stimulated by adrenaline secretion that accelerates heartbeat so that the heart pumps more blood into the muscles. At the end of a period of physical activity, endorphins are released and give your body a feeling of wellbeing and relaxation.

This also explains why various clinical studies indicate that exercise helps reduce anxiety, stress and depressive symptoms, and this also has a beneficial effect on acne.

Moderate and regular physical activity also helps reduce fat mass, improve sugars meabolism and decrease insulin secretion, reducing the overall and acne inflammation status.

Finally, it strengthens the immune system.

While you exercise, there is also an intense sweating that helps to expel toxins. However, in some cases, in people with sensitive skin, it may also aggravate pimples due to skin irritation.

You should therefore avoid synthetic and tight clothing, regularly wipe sweat off your face and take a shower immediately after your workout.

In order to get all the benefits from exercising, you do not need to go to the gym every day or go for intensive workouts; this might actually be counterproductive because it seems to stimulate greater production of male hormones.

To relax and oxygenate better, you only need to walk 30 minutes a day, possibly outdoors and in fresh air, or do gentle gym sessions or dance to combine physical activity and fun.

HEALTHY FUN
Relax and have fun

Real fun should be enjoyable and satisfy us deeply. Its main feature is participation and the game itself: dancing, laughing and joking with friends without necessarily "feeling high".

There are so many activities that can naturally give us satisfaction, either done alone or with somebody else: whether it is a walk in the city or on the seashore, a football, basketball or volleyball match, or even a videogame.

The important thing is that it should "engage" us so much that we would disregard any other things and totally enjoy that precise moment: this is the so-called "flow" experience described by psychologists.

When we are in the "flow", our mind is intensely concentrated, but relaxed at the same time: even in this case, our brain produces endorphins and gives us wellbeing and happiness, balancing the whole hormone system and freeing us from stress and inflammation.

HEALTHY ATTITUDE
Perseverance, patience and trust

I earlier mentioned that a happier life leads us to achieve our goals more easily, improves our health and our psycho-physical wellbeing, but also the opposite is true: setting and achieving our goals, taking care of our health and trying to feel as good as possible with ourselves makes our life more beautiful and happier.

This establishes a positive cycle that strengthens over time and becomes a lifestyle.

However, now I want to warn you about a great obstacle that you might encounter on the path you want to undertake or that you have already begun through the advice of this book. You will soon discover how the pursuit of perfection is a boulder on the path of your freedom from pimples and on the path of your happiness.

There is difference between struggling for the best result and aiming for total perfection. The first attitude has an achievable goal and is gratifying and healthy; the second has an often unachievable goal and is frustrating and a source of neurosis. Furthermore, it involves an absurd waste of time.
(Edwin Bliss, journalist)

Aiming for perfection to improve and improve the world around us and wanting perfection in everything and at any cost are two apparently similar attitudes, but with very different effects.

Perfectionism, the pursuit of perfection at all costs, is a real trap.

If you are not perfect and do not get perfect results, you will never have self-esteem and respect for yourself, and you will never be happy.

Any small mistake or setback causes frustration, fierce self-criticism and a feeling of failure: do you remember what you read about self-esteem and motivation in the first two steps?

If you want to have a perfect face without a single pimple, but you do not accept that – despite good improvement or normalisation of your skin – every now and then some pimple may appear, you are condemning yourself to useless stress and suffering and, probably, to a further worsening of your acne.

Moreover, you will never be satisfied, if you look at each situation (and yourself) by comparing it with an absolute perfection that will never be achievable for a simple reason: it does not exist in the real world!

Perfect people do not fight, do not lie, do not make mistakes and do not exist.
(Aristotle)

And if you try and reach perfection, you will just waste your time! If you think about it, this is the trap: an alibi for not trying or not taking action, because you know that you will never achieve the ideal goal.

Think about it, you cannot reason bluntly: perfect or nothing. Here, realising that there is a middle ground in every situation and perfection does not exist leads us to the concept of possibility and flexibility.

In achieving a goal or in pursuit of perfection while knowing it is unachievable, we can progress step by step through a continuous improvement, with the necessary flexibility, ready to change our route or strategy in case of unavoidable obstacles and setbacks.

Even when you cure acne you should take into account these concepts:
- perfectionism as a mental block (or as an alibi for doing nothing or giving up)
- accepting that reality is made of steps forwards and backwards;
- the right flexibility in order to change therapeutic strategy
- acknowledgement and satisfaction in achieving intermediate goals.

When you aim for perfection, you discover it is a moving target.
(George Fisher, writer)

Indeed, **in order to keep yourself away from perfectionism mania**, you should:

- set goals by taking into account what is really possible, based on your circumstances, capabilities and means – always trying to progress, with patience and detachment,

- know that it is not always possible to reach a goal immediately and fully, that there are ups and downs, and that sometimes you will be forced to go backwards, but you will then move forward.

The secret is to accept life, circumstances and yourself with flexibility.

Perfection is not perfect, but continuously striving for it.
(Johann Gottlieb Fichte, philosopher)

THE PURSUIT OF HAPPINESS

Success does not mean the absence of failures. It means the attainment of ultimate objectives.
(Edwin Bliss, writer)

The ultimate goal of improving your physical appearance is the ability to like yourself, to be liked by others and to be happy.

The pursuit of happiness is the fundamental goal of each of us, but we often cannot explain what happiness is and we really do not know how to find it.

Indeed, not feeling and seeing your face full of pimples, or even better, having healthy and clean skin, and a face free from acne is a source of psychological wellbeing and more relaxed and pleasant social relations. However, it is important to realise that linking the achievement happiness to the absence of pimples is very similar to the trap of perfectionism.

Happiness is a state to strive for, which is favoured by so many other factors including that of having a pleasant physical appearance.

The paradox is that being happy can also improve the state of our skin thanks to all the complex psycho-neuro-immune-endocrine influences that I have repeatedly referred to in this book.

This is the goal of the whole path: treating skin well and winning against acne in order to find balance, maturity, strength, wellbeing and happiness; and being strong and happy to improve the beauty of your own skin and self.

Michael Fordyce, psychologist and pioneer in pursuit of happiness, has thoroughly studied the features that characterise happy people from those who are not.

It has been shown that a person can learn to be happier when he/she has these attitudes.

They can lead to significant changes in behaviours, and therefore in daily life and in the way of approaching the world, by favouring a change in our beliefs (…and possibilities).

I want to conclude this chapter on lifestyle with the Fordyce's 14 characteristics of happy people, partially reworded by me:

- Be active and keep yourself busy: cultivate your interests, follow your passions.
- Spend more time socialising: surrounded by people you appreciate and vice versa.
- Be more productive by doing meaningful activities: have a purpose in life.
- Organise yourself at best and set goals: be organised.
- Stop worrying: accept the ups and downs of life.
- Live life with detachment: accept imperfection.
- Develop positive thoughts and be optimistic: always see the glass half full.
- Be oriented to the present: live consciously.
- Work on a healthy personality: constantly improve yourself.
- Develop a sociable character: be altruistic.
- Be yourself: respect yourself and your uniqueness.
- Eliminate negative feelings and problems: distinguish the problems that you can solve.
- Be able to identify with others: respect the others.
- Consider happiness as a fundamental priority: apply these principles.

THE ACNE SIGNS: HOW TO PREVENT AND IMPROVE THEM

ACNE SPOTS

How many times you have seen your overall skin's status progressively improving, pimples dry up and become less inflamed in no time without leaving holes and scars... but, unfortunately, where there were papules and pustules, you notice evident red and brown spots. Even after several days or months, they are still there and did not even fade a little.

Even when acne does not leave permanent signs such as post-acne scarring, it can leave residues that tend to last for a long time and look like blemishes, thus cancelling the benefits of the treatments – in the patient's eyes.

We can distinguish **two different types of spots**:

1. dark or brown spots from post-inflammatory hyperpigmentation.
2. post-inflammatory red spots.

Post-inflammatory spots are a persistent inflammatory process associated with pimples.

They can be determined by various factors:

- the phototype (there is a higher probability in those who have olive or brown skin),
- exposure to sunlight or sun lamps, traumatic actions on pimples (picking and squeezing),
- the use of photosensitizing anti-acne antibiotics (such as tetracyclines) when exposed to the sun.

Red spots are the residue of the acneic inflammatory process that gradually, but very slowly, vanishes over time, generally ranging from 15 days to 2-3 months. There is a vasodilation in the surface and medium dermis that tends to be persistent.

What can we do to eliminate these unhealthy spots that remain after the pimples?

Let us start by saying that in most cases they are almost a natural evolution of the pimple: during the slow healing and repair process of the skin around and at the level of the pimple, the inflammatory substances stimulate vasodilation and melanocytes to produce melanin in excess.

Therefore, as for acne scars, it would be better to prevent acne spots because they are more difficult to treat.

We should then always try to avoid excessive inflammation of the pimples with inadequate cure or aggressive picking and squeezing and, in any case, accelerate healing:

the sooner the pimples dry out and become less inflamed, the better.

Generally, with some chemical peeling sessions, you can obtain this result quickly.

Peeling is also useful in eliminating acne spots more rapidly because, paradoxically, its irritating, cauterising and stimulating action on the dermis facilitates repair and normalisation. Even if immediate inflammation and vasodilation increases the redness and burning, it then resets and extinguishes the acneic inflammatory process, so the red spots from pimples visibly fade and brown spots improve – although this is achievable more gradually.

Overall, the skin becomes clearer, brighter and cleaner.

ACNE SCARS

In most cases, the face is the area most affected by acne and therefore also by acne scars. The face is our business card, the most visible part of our body; it is our identity.

This often leads patients with acne scars to have significant difficulties in interpersonal relationships: this can aggravate psychological problems that are often already present because of pimples, sometimes causing social isolation and severe depression.

The risk of pimples leaving scars should therefore be a strong motivation to timely undergo a dermatological examination and regularly follow the recommended home-based therapy and outpatient treatments.

In fact, an adequate care is essential to prevent permanent damage caused by acne.

Once the scars have formed, the patient and the dermatologist specialist face different treatment options to improve the appearance of the skin: these choices are based on the type of scars and on the patient's expectations.

There are basically two types of acne scars:
1.   **prominent** or **hypertrophic** or **keloid**
2.   **depressed** or **atrophic**

The former are less frequent and have a rosy or dark red colour.
They are due to an excessive or abnormal scarring process as a response to the destruction of deep dermis: fibrous tissue production does not block on its own as it happens in normal wound repair.
There is often a particular predisposition at the basis, scars are often a complication of isotretinoin therapy.

In these cases, it is possible to react with various treatments, including the most traditional (but cheap and effective) sessions of intralesional cortisone injections, possibly combined with cryotherapy, which reduce and block the formation of fibrous tissue.
The scar gradually decreases in volume and height. The number of sessions is variable and depends on the lesion response.

Depressed scars are the most common and their depth depends on the severity and depth of the inflammation process that has occurred.

They can be:
- **superficial** (they are almost similar to spots), with slightly reddened or hyperpigmented bottom,
- **deep**, 1-2 mm diameter with sharp edges (looking like small holes) or up to 1-2 cm diameter with shaded edges (looking like craters): if they are numerous, crater-shaped lesions can look noticeably disfiguring, representing a serious blemish.

Is it possible to prevent hole-shaped acne scars?

These skin lesions look like small holes with sharp edges and have various depths. If they are very small, they can be confused with dilated pores. These scars have formed for a loss of dermal tissue. The dermis faced destruction during the pimple inflammatory process manifested in the form of papules, pustules or nodules. Generally, papules and pustules cause point-shaped depressed scars, but the nodule is deeper and bigger, and causes crater-shaped depressed acne scars.

Pus contains white blood cells that release inflammatory substances and enzymes that corrode and destroy the skin, leaving scars.

Because of their small diameter and depth, correcting scars can be difficult, that is why you should prevent them by:

- Treating acne from the beginning following the dermatologist's therapy before it becomes more serious. It may sound obvious but I have seen many cases where the patients tried to treat pimples by themselves, making attempts that led to no benefits or even a worsening: the only result was the formation of scars.
- Never squeezing the pimple or undergo traumatic facial cleansing.
- Gently stinging the initial or "mature" pustules with a sterile needle to let the pus come out without forcing, and then apply an antibiotic gel recommended by the dermatologist.
- In the case of pustule acne on the face, following antibiotic treatments via general administration or undergoing chemical peeling with salicylic acid or trichloroacetic acid in order to rapidly dry out pustules and pimples.

How to improve acne scars

You might think, or some educational or promotional articles might want us to think, that acne holes and scars can be eliminated more easily, perhaps with a miraculous session of the last laser released on the market.

You should not delude yourself, correcting all scars has limits: it is important to understand that, unfortunately, **you cannot erase them**.

What you can do is improve their appearance, making them less visible. Their visibility is a matter of optics: the deeper they are, the greater is the shadow projected on the bottom or the surrounding skin (this also depends on the incidence of the light. In fact, we can all see how the visibility of any alteration of the skin surface i.e. wrinkles, scars or the like varies depending on the lighting of the environment or how we move the head in relation to the light source, be it from the sun or artificial).

Therefore, we can get an improvement either by reducing the raised part of the hypertrophic scars (as we have seen before) or lowering the edges of those depressed or, again, lifting the bottom of skin depression.

Camouflage or **corrective make-up** tends to mask imperfections, darker or redder areas, using neutralising colours (e.g. green on red) or lightening. The bottom of the scar is made clearer so that the shadow is less dark and evident. In this case, however, there is only an apparent improvement, but not a permanent one.

There are also the different corrective techniques of aesthetic dermatology that can be integrated into a treatment programme in order to obtain the best possible result.

We can generally classify them as resurfacing or levelling techniques, filling techniques, and surgical correction techniques.

Resurfacing techniques tend to smooth the skin surface by levelling it.

Among these, one of the first to be used was **dermabrasion**, which consists of the mechanical abrasion of the skin by a diamond fraise. If there is a large number of lesions, it is advisable to abrade a large area or entire face. It is an aggressive method that improves very deep scars, regardless of their width.

Another procedure is the superficial and medium-depth **chemical peeling**: in this case, the smoothing effect is given by one or more acidic substances (trichloroacetic acid, phenol) which destroy the epidermis and part of the dermis. This technique is less aggressive than dermabrasion, and after a variable number of sessions, it results in a visible and sharp improvement in the slightly depressed (superficial macular) scars; for more severe scars, it is not enough on its own. Even **fractional laser** and **fractional radiofrequency** have a smoothing effect on the skin, improving the edges of depressed scars.

The **filling techniques** consist of implanting substances (via microinjection) in the dermis in order to lift the bottom of the scar and bring it to the level of the healthy surrounding skin. These substances are generally collagen-based materials, hyaluronic acid or adipose tissue of the patient (they are the ones that give fewer complications even if they have the disadvantage only being temporarily beneficial: the duration is variable from subject to subject and the treatment needs to be repeated).

Lifting the bottom, the height of the vertical walls of the scar consequently decreases: the shadow projection will be minor so that the crater will appear less noticeable.

Hyaluronic acid injections not only produce a fill, hyaluronic acid does much more! It has a biorevitalising and stimulating effect on the dermis that determines to a new collagen production, leading to a certain degree of permanent improvement of the scar, which becomes progressive with periodic repetition of the treatment.

Finally, we have various **surgical correction techniques**:
- subcision, where a needle with a sharp blade is inserted into the skin to cut the scarring attachments that cause the surface of the skin to dimple (very useful for the crater-shaped acne and varicella scars as well as post-traumatic scars),
- surgical micro excision via special cylindrical scalpel,
- the surgical lifting of the scar up to the level of the surrounding skin,
- skin transplantation, in which the surgically removed scar is replaced by a portion of skin taken from the back of the ears.

They are very suitable for crater-shaped and sharp-edged depressed scars, although the result is not always the best, but it depends very much on post-treatment progress and dermal response.

According to my experience, you can really obtain good results using the **subcision** technique I mentioned above: it consists of using a very thin needle to remove the adhesions between the scar (or wrinkle) and the underlying deep tissue. This treatment is much less challenging than others, but generally cheaper and more effective – perhaps, that is why it is little advertised.

During the same session, small amounts of hyaluronic acid can possibly be injected under the scar.

In this way, we gain greater benefits:
1. removal of adhesions
2. lifting of the bottom of the scar
3. the formation of a hyaluronic acid pad under the scar, to further lift the bottom and support it

4. biorevitalisation of the skin around and under the scar with new collagen formation
5. partial, but progressive and permanent correction of the scar.

In fact, if you repeat the treatment at regular intervals based on the response of your skin, you will then get a gradual correction of crater-shaped or hole-shaped depressed scars.

For crater-shaped scars, the results are better and faster.

In order to achieve further improvement, treatments to smooth the skin and the edges of the scars can be performed (e.g. peeling and fractional radiofrequency).

All outpatient treatments described must always be performed by an expert dermatologist as they are not free from risks or complications. It is then important to understand that the scars correction process needs to be gradual and well planned (it takes at least a few months) and finally, it is always necessary to combine the various methods in order to achieve the best aesthetic benefits possible.

IN CONCLUSION

If you have reached this point, you have probably done the tests and exercises suggested, and you are on the right track to effectively fight pimples. Now you should have all the data and clear ideas to act quickly.

From now on, use the 7 steps method daily – as an encouragement to finally keep yourself on track and not to lose yourself along the way.

I hope this book is useful to you: it does not contain quick remedies for pimples or promises of miracles, you cannot get there without the dermatologist's advice and dermatological care, but will certainly help you to change your approach to pimples treatment and your lifestyle.

It will inspire you and guide you, motivate you to do something really important and meaningful to you and your life.

Indeed, treating acne properly will bring you to improve your image, your self-esteem and your social relations.

DID YOU LIKE THIS BOOK?
Writing a review will let other people know about it.

And do not forget to follow me on social networks:

https://www.facebook.com/DermatologiaCosmetologica
https://www.google.com/+DermatologiaCosmetologicalT
https://www.google.com/+dottFrancescoAntonaccioParma
https://twitter.com/Dermocosmetolog

APPENDIX A
HOW TO READ THE LABELS OF COSMETIC PRODUCTS

by Dr Beatrice De Carne, cosmetic chemist and responsible for the cosmetology section of our blog.

It is important to know how to read the label of cosmetic products in order to have a grasp of its composition: indeed, we apply cosmetic products to our skin every day. They contain different chemical substances and it is good to know what we are using, if their molecules are valid and present in appropriate concentration. However, the composition of a cosmetic product is not always understandable because of the nomenclature used to identify the ingredients, the so-called INCI.

The INCI, International Nomenclature of Cosmetic Ingredients, defines an international and standard denomination of each ingredient used in the cosmetic field.

Some ingredients may have different INCIs in Europe, France and the USA.

First rule:
By law, each cosmetic product indicates the complete list of ingredients in descending order of concentration up to 1%.

How to read the INCI of cosmetic products and recognise the ingredients? In most cosmetics, the first component of the list is water as it is present at higher concentrations. In Europe, water is identified by the INCI name of Latin origin aqua, while water and eau are respectively the American and French INCIs. These INCIs are on the label only if the product is marketed in those countries. Alcohol Denat, instead, is the INCI of ethyl alcohol (common alcohol) that can be used in cosmetics as a solvent (especially in hair products), antiseptic or to improve cream texture.

In cosmetics, other ingredients with the INCI containing the word alcohol are used, but they are compounds totally different from ethyl alcohol, in fact they are generally fatty substances such as cetearyl alcohol (widely used to give consistency to creams).

Second rule:
Natural substances are easily identifiable: their INCI contains the Latin name of the plant from which they originate (e.g. olive oil = olea europaea), followed by the English name of the part of the plant utilised (root, leaf, fruit) and the product typology (oil, extract, water).

For instance, the full INCI for olive oil: olea europaea fruit oil.

The identification of structural substances (such as emulsifiers, consistency factors and emollients) is more complex.

These are components that do not have any kind of biological function, but they are utilised to formulate specific product types such as creams, milks, gels, oils, etc. They are used with concentrations above 1%, so they are found in the upper or middle part of the label.

Third rule:
The INCI of structural substances is represented by the corresponding chemical name which, in most cases, is not immediately understood.

Fourth rule:
The INCIs functional substances are many and different depending on the type of ingredient employed.

Certain functional substances are easily recognisable by their partial name found in the INCI: it is the case of sodium hyaluronate which identifies hyaluronic acid or peptides as acetyl hexapeptide-9.

Other functional substances may be less identifiable as they are indicated by their chemical name.

Vitamins are a typical example: tocopherol is the INCI of vitamin E, retinyl palmitate or retinol represents the INCI of vitamin A and retinol respectively. In these cases, you can also examine the description of claims and action of active ingredients present on the packaging.

And silicones? Methicone or siloxane are part of the INCI for most silicones; this category includes a wide range of compounds with different functionalities and can be used at different percentages, so they do not have a very precise place in the label.

Fifth rule:
At the bottom of the ingredients list, you will find preservatives, colours and perfumes because they are used with concentrations of less than 1%.

In cosmetic products, preservatives are needed to preserve the product microbiologically: they are indicated by their chemical name to better identify their structure. It is known that some may be the cause of sensitisation, irritation or allergies to those more predisposed. In waterless products or in those with a high content of denaturated alcohol, preservatives are absent.

Colours are identified by the CI, color index, followed by a 5-digit number defining the colour tone.

Perfumes are indicated with the European and American INCI, respectively perfume or fragrance. However, this name is not exhaustive because the composition of a perfume includes some ingredients (including essential oils) which are potential allergens – they are indeed indicated on the label for consumer protection. Among these allergens, the most present is limonene. To date, the only exception is the essential oil of patchouli that does not contain allergens.

COMEDOGENIC SUBSTANCES:

Butyl stearate
Cocoa butter
Corn oil
D&C red dyes
Decyl oleate
Isopropyl isostearate
Isopropyl myristate
Isopropyl neopenatanate
Isopropyl palmitate
Isopropyl stearate
Lanolin acetylated
Linseed oil
Laureth-4
Mineral oil
Myristyl ether propionate
Myristyl lactate
Myristyl myristate
Oleic acid
Oleyl alcohol
Olive oil
Octyl palmitate

Octyl stearate
Peanut oil
Methyl oleate
Petrolatum (paraffin o vaseline)
Safflower oil
Sesame oil
Sodium lauryl sulphate
Stearic acid

THE AUTHOR

Francesco Antonaccio MD, is dermatologist, creator and founder of the website Dermatologia Cosmetologica: Benessere e Cura della Pelle.

He has focused his dermatologist's work on the study and treatment of facial skin imperfections for years, and is an expert in acne and anti-aging treatments.

He attended and has attended Courses and Congresses as tutor and lecturer.

He lives and works in Parma - Italy.

OTHER AUTHOR'S BOOKS:

**Curare Rosacea Couperose e Pelle sensibile:
le 3 azioni chiave per curare la pelle sensibile**

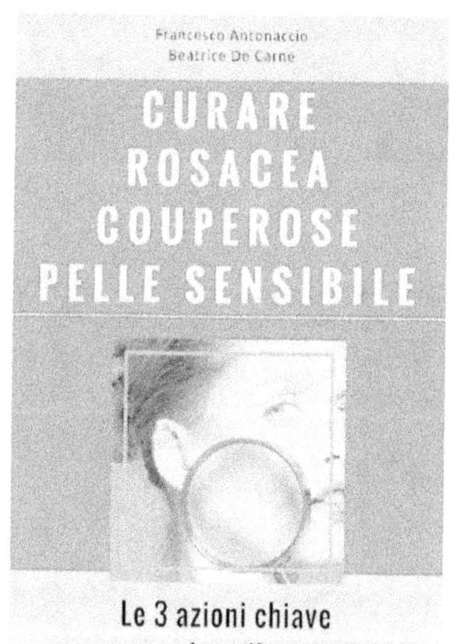

www.ingramcontent.com/pod-product-compliance
Lightning Source LLC
Chambersburg PA
CBHW050805260726

48660CB00004B/1259